Justin Derwent grew up in Yorkshire and qualified in dentistry at Leeds University. Later he studied for a Master's degree in medical law at Cardiff University. He now lives with his wife and their ever-increasing family of animals in an old farmhouse on the Dorset/Somerset border.

Also by Justin Derwent:

Practice Makes Perfect

TEETHING TROUBLES

To my very good friend, Roger, who was an integral part of my early days in general dental practice.

TEETHING
TROUBLES

by

JUSTIN DERWENT

CHAPTER ONE

A sudden blast of cold air swept through the entrance hall as the front door was almost wrenched from its hinges. It crashed open against the inside wall and the wrought iron handle gouged a depression in the soft lime plaster. A lumbering figure which looked every bit as big and solid as the steel-studded oak door seemed to fill the entire opening. His red hair was on end and his piercing blue eyes blazed with anger.

'Where's Derwent?' he bellowed as he leapt forward into the hall.

Beryl was unfortunate enough to be the one he addressed and immediately wondered whether her job description, if she had one, would state that she would be required to deal with this sort of encounter.

'I want to see Derwent, now,' the man roared.

'*Mr* Derwent is with a patient at the moment,' said Beryl softly, 'but I'll tell him you want to see him if you give me your name. Would you like to take a seat in the waiting room?'

The man approached Beryl and she recoiled as the breath emanating from his mouth and nostrils scalded her face like superheated steam. His breathing was rapid and shallow. 'No, I wouldn't – I demand to see him now. Either you go and fetch him this minute or I'll go and drag him out here myself.'

'I'll go and tell him you're anxious to see him,' said Beryl calmly, hoping that a gentle response might encourage him to cool down, 'but he can't just leave his patient in the middle of treatment. I'm sure he'll see you as soon as he can. Have you a problem?'

'Do I have a problem? A problem? That's a bloody understatement – I've got a problem all right and it's his fault. Now go and get him because I'm getting very impatient.'

'Who shall I say wants to see him?'

'Just go and fetch him!'

'Can I have your name?'

'Newman.'

'Are you a patient of his?'

'I've seen him once but this is not about me; it's about my wife but I can tell you that by the time I've finished with him he'll be in no fit state to treat any patients for some time.'

'Please take a seat, Mr Newman. I'll go and tell him you want to see him.'

She scuttled off to my surgery as quickly as possible leaving Mr Newman thrashing around in the entrance hall like a wild animal poised to pounce on its prey.

'There's a Mr Newman in the hall demanding to see you, Justin. He seems very angry about something; in fact, he's quite threatening.'

'Mr Newman? I don't think I know him. Oh yes, it must be Mrs Newman's husband. Do you know why he wants to see me?'

'No, he didn't say but he's fuming about something. He's very aggressive and I think you need to be careful because he seems intent on doing you harm for some reason.'

I was in no mood for a confrontation but I was obviously going to have to find out what was troubling him. I was about to say that I would go to see him as soon as I finished with my patient but Mr Newman had a different idea – he was already banging on the door of my surgery with a huge clenched fist.

He lunged towards me like a rampaging bull and for a moment I thought he was going to trample me into the floor but he stopped short once he was within arm's length and his enormous left hand closed around my throat. Towering above me by at least twelve inches he pushed me backwards until my shoulder blades thudded against the surgery door. His right index finger was like the barrel of a twelve bore prodding me in the ribs.

'Because of you, my wife's left me,' he hollered. 'Twelve years we've been married, twelve years! Everything was fine until you came on the scene and got your hands on her. You've a hell of a lot to answer for. What have you got to say for yourself?.... Eh?..... Eh?'

CHAPTER TWO

'You look pleased with yourself, Spencer,' I remarked as I went into the office to grab a quick cup of coffee. The morning had already presented me with more than my fair share of problems and I felt in need of some refreshment before facing the next patient. Beryl was typing and Spencer was sitting by the window, with his feet on the desk, reading the Times.

'As a matter of fact I am,' he replied. 'I had a phone call last night from the daughter of Lady Gascoyne-Fairley.' He paused as if to give me time to assimilate the significance of this statement.

'Am I supposed to know who Lady Gascoyne-Fairley is?' I enquired.

'Justin, I am sometimes astounded by your ignorance of the world. Sir Richard Gascoyne-Fairley is hugely famous. He is a highly successful businessman who has built up an amazing reputation for taking struggling businesses and turning them into multimillion-pound organizations. Naturally, he is enormously wealthy and owns a large country mansion and estate not far from here, where he and Lady Gascoyne-Fairley spend much of the summer. If you take the road to the coast from here you'll pass the entrance to the estate; it's on the right hand side of the road about two miles from the town centre. I must admit I haven't heard much about him recently; he's probably getting on a bit in age now and may have slowed down his business activities, but people like that never really retire.'

'I regret to say I've never heard of him. But why did the daughter phone you?'

'It seems that Lady Gascoyne-Fairley needs a dentist. She hasn't had any treatment for many years because she hates dentistry, but she's now starting to get pain and has finally accepted that she'll need to face getting her teeth sorted out. According to her daughter, she's likely to need a whole load of work done and they want me to do it. It will, of course, be private and I'm sure the cost will be of no concern to them whatsoever.'

'I get it. You see a cash register before your very eyes. No wonder you look pleased with yourself.'

'No, no, no, Justin. It's not like that at all. I see this as an indication that my practice is getting the recognition it deserves. My reputation is spreading and I'm beginning to attract a better class of patient. Who knows where this could lead? Sir Richard and Lady Gascoyne-Fairley are bound to have lots of very important and wealthy friends and these people talk. As long as I make a good impression on her I don't see how I can fail to attract some very desirable new private patients.'

'So when is she coming?'

'At about eleven o'clock this morning. I said not to worry too much if they can't get here dead on time.'

'What about your other patients? Your morning was already booked wasn't it?'

'As soon as I finished speaking to Lady Gascoyne-Fairley's daughter I got Daphne to cancel everyone from ten-thirty onwards so that I would have the rest of the morning clear. Beryl has ordered some fresh flowers for the entrance hall and waiting room; not that I intend to keep Lady Gascoyne-Fairley waiting for more than a few moments, but I want everywhere to look bright and cheerful. I've also arranged for Mrs Crossley to stay on an hour longer this morning to make sure the whole place is spotlessly clean. Who have you got coming in after eleven o'clock?'

'Mr and Mrs Edmondson for their check-ups, and Mr Wiltshire for some fillings.'

'That should be all right; they are respectable enough. I wouldn't want there to be any noisy children in the waiting room, or anyone who might spoil the image of the practice in any way.'

'That's a terrible thing to say, Spencer. They're all patients and they all deserve to be treated with respect.'

'Oh absolutely, Justin, you're quite right. It's just that I feel that first impressions are very important and I don't want anything to go wrong. If I can win over Lady Gascoyne-Fairley it could prove enormously beneficial to the future of the practice.'

Ingrid came in to tell me that my next patient had arrived so I went back to my surgery taking my cup of coffee with me.

Eleven o'clock arrived and so far there was no sign of Spencer's very important patient. I was aware that he was pacing around like an expectant father. He had put on a freshly laundered white overall and kept going to the window to see if there was any sign of an expensive car arriving.

At about twenty-five past eleven a taxi pulled into the drive of the practice and a smartly dressed, middle-aged woman emerged from the offside rear door. She walked round to the other side of the taxi and was immediately joined by the driver. Neither of them was aware that Spencer, Beryl and Ingrid had their noses pressed to the upstairs window watching intently.

'She's arrived,' announced Ingrid as she returned to my surgery to help me with my patients.

'So you know about Lady Grasping-Firmly or whatever she's called?' I quipped somewhat cynically. I couldn't help thinking that this whole business had served to put Spencer in one of his more pompous moods and there was a good chance things would not turn out be quite as rosy as he was hoping.

'Lady Gascoyne-Fairley,' Ingrid corrected, 'and yes, Beryl told me all about her. Spencer is very excited about it.'

'I know. I just hope it doesn't end in tears.'

'Why should it?' said Ingrid.

'No reason, I just hope it doesn't that's all. Did you see her?'

'I just caught a glimpse of her as they tried to get her out of the taxi. She isn't exactly young and she is quite …well, big.'

Mr Edmondson was sitting in my dental chair waiting for me to check his teeth and although he didn't seem to be paying the slightest attention to our conversation, I decided it was unethical to be discussing another patient in his presence. I said no more about Lady Gascoyne-Fairley and Ingrid handed me a mouth mirror and a probe so that I could get on with examining his teeth.

I barely had time to look at the first molar when Beryl burst into my surgery in something of a panic. 'Justin, can you and Ingrid come right away and help us with Lady Gascoyne-Fairley? She isn't very good on her legs and we are having great difficulty getting her up the stairs.'

'I am sorry about this Mr Edmondson,' I said. 'Will you excuse us for a few moments? There appears to be a problem.'

'That's all right,' he replied. 'I'm not in any hurry.'

As we got to the top of the stairs Spencer called out furiously, 'Quick, Justin, come and give me a hand, I can't hold her much longer.'

Lady Gascoyne-Fairley, although extremely elderly, was by no means a lightweight. She had reached the third tread of the staircase and Spencer was crouching down behind her, propping her up to prevent her from falling back down the stairs and she appeared to be sitting on his left shoulder. Lady Gascoyne-Fairley's companion who was, in fact, her daughter was at the foot of the stairs and her resolute stance with her hands on her hips indicated that she had no intention of playing any part in the operation to elevate her mother to the first floor.

I ran down the stairs to help but it was difficult to know what to do. The combined bulk of Lady Gascoyne-Fairley and Spencer blocked the entire width of the stairs preventing me from getting past them and, quite clearly, it was motive force from behind that was required to propel her upwards.

'Quick, grab her arms,' shrieked Spencer whose face was turning an intense shade of crimson with the effort. 'I can't hold her.'

I took her right hand and Ingrid seized her left and we both tugged for all our might. Our efforts successfully dislodged her from Spencer's shoulder but unfortunately the pull was rather too enthusiastic and Lady Gascoyne-Fairley lurched forwards and was in danger of falling flat on her face. Spencer saw what was happening and was quick to compensate by throwing his arm around her neck to restrain her. He managed to stabilize her but the position of his arm was such that a casual observer could be excused for thinking he was trying to strangle her. The scream let out by Lady Gascoyne-Fairley suggested that she had come to a similar conclusion. He released his grip and she swayed back and forth for a few moments before her knees began to buckle. Ingrid and I saved her from crumpling altogether by supporting her under her elbows.

We held her firmly, wondering what the next move would be and Spencer composed himself after his previous exertions. He was obviously wondering the same thing.

'You lift her by her arms and I'll take the weight from behind,' he gasped, 'and we'll walk her upstairs a step at a time.'

In order to support her from behind Spencer put his hands under her shoulder blades and whilst this prevented her from falling backwards it was ineffective in providing the necessary uplift. He had no alternative, therefore, but to shift his grasp to somewhere under her buttocks.

Apart from the indignity, it seemed a reasonable plan but for some reason Lady Gascoyne-Fairley suddenly became afflicted with a sort of rigor. Her feet were leaden and her legs became as stiff as gateposts. No amount of persuasion, coercion, pushing, pulling or lifting could advance a single foot on to the next tread.

'It's no good,' Spencer wheezed. 'We aren't getting anywhere like this. We're going to have to carry her. Beryl, you come and help.'

Lady Gascoyne-Fairley's daughter, who still hadn't lifted a finger to offer assistance, was becoming increasingly edgy. 'This is ridiculous,' she sneered. 'Why didn't you tell me the surgery was upstairs? I wouldn't have brought her here if I'd known. You can see she isn't capable of climbing stairs.'

'Don't worry,' said Spencer reassuringly, desperate to uphold an image of calm efficiency in spite of the present dilemma. 'We're used to helping patients like your mother up and down stairs. Beryl and Ingrid, you take a leg each and, Justin, you come down here with me and we'll carry her by her arms.'

Thus it was that Lady Gascoyne-Fairley's considerable weight was hoisted one step at a time up the stairs and finally dumped in a disbelieving and dishevelled heap on the landing by four very breathless and relieved members of the Spencer Padginton dental practice. For some time no-one moved except Lady Gascoyne-Fairley's daughter who came up the stairs to join us. 'How the hell are you going to get her back down again?' she demanded.

'Don't worry about that,' Spencer responded steadily. 'It'll be easier because gravity will be in our favour.'

Ingrid and I shared glances and I saw her struggle to suppress a smirk. I am sure her thoughts and mine were similar and we pictured a somewhat out of control descent of the stairs with Lady Gascoyne-Fairley's weight providing the kinetic energy to convey her back to the ground floor, with Spencer hanging on to her for dear life in order to moderate the speed of descent.

When everyone had recovered their composure, the four of us surrounded the patient and manhandled her into Spencer's surgery where we thankfully deposited her in his dental chair. Ingrid and I returned to my surgery where Mr Edmondson was still waiting, completely oblivious to everything that had been going on.

Spencer was with Lady Gascoyne-Fairley for about three quarters of an hour before Ingrid and I were summoned once again to assist in getting her back downstairs. Spencer's prediction that it would be easier going down, fortunately, turned out to be true and was greatly assisted by the fact that some of the use in her legs had apparently returned, so she wasn't quite the deadweight she had been previously. Spencer and I held her by the arms, and Ingrid took up position immediately in front of Lady Gascoyne-Fairley, theoretically to block her in case she should fall forwards, though on reflection I think it was most unlikely that the nurse's slender frame would have succeeded in holding back the considerable weight of the distinguished patient.

We installed her in the waiting room and Beryl phoned for a taxi to come and pick her up. After I had finished seeing Mr and Mrs Edmondson I sought out Spencer to find out how he had got on with his titled patient.

'Pretty well,' I think. 'She and I seemed to hit it off from the start. It seems we have a lot of similar interests. We are both very keen on opera and ballet.'

'Are you, Spencer? You've never mentioned it before.'

'Haven't I? Oh yes I love opera and ballet, particularly opera.'

'When did you last go to the opera?'

Spencer looked a little ruffled by my probing but maintained his composure. 'Well it is some time ago, I must admit, but that's because I'm so busy doing other things and of course, one has to travel some considerable distance to find good opera so it isn't easy when you are running a busy dental practice.'

'No, of course not.' I decided to change the subject. 'Anyway how did her treatment go?'

'Oh extremely well, though I didn't do an awful lot. We spent most of the time talking. I felt it was better for us to get to know each other before embarking on any real dental treatment. Establishing a good relationship with patients is very important.'

'I know it is but she came to see you because she had toothache, didn't she?'

'She's had a bit of pain but I don't think it's anything too serious. I gave her some painkillers and antibiotics, which should help in the short term.'

'Did you carry out a full examination?'

'Well, no not really. I had a quick look to get an overall impression of the state of her teeth and to establish the likely cause of her trouble but she isn't very keen on having treatment. I had to tread very carefully at this stage. I don't want to frighten her off, do I?'

'So it wasn't all that profitable for you then if you didn't do any treatment?'

'Justin, you still have an awful lot to learn about the treatment of private patients. Lady Gascoyne-Fairley has sought my professional services and my time. I shall, therefore, be charging her for my time at a rate which reflects the level of my expertise. The amount of actual dentistry carried out is irrelevant.'

'That all sounds good in theory,' I scoffed, 'but she did, after all, come to you to get dental treatment. Don't you think she might get a bit upset if you put in a huge bill when all you actually did was to have a quick look in her mouth and give her some tablets?'

'Of course she won't get upset. Apart from the fact that money is no object, people like Lady Gascoyne-Fairley don't seek professional services from someone without first checking them out thoroughly so they can be a hundred percent sure they can trust them implicitly. This means she'll accept my way of doing things without question.'

'They couldn't have checked you out all that thoroughly; they didn't even know your surgery was upstairs. Her daughter said she wouldn't have come here if she'd known.'

'That's different. I'm talking about my treatment and my professional skills.'

'Presumably you'll be seeing a lot more of her so how are you going to get round the problem of getting her upstairs each time?'

'Oh don't worry we'll manage somehow. We got her upstairs today, didn't we?'

'It was a bit of a struggle. I'm sure none of us, particularly Lady Gascoyne-Fairley wants to go through that every time she comes here.'

'Don't concern yourself, Justin, just leave it to me; I'll sort it out.'

CHAPTER THREE

'I've got something to tell you, Justin,' Ingrid announced hesitantly.

'Why do I get the feeling I'm not going to like what you are about to tell me?'

Ingrid sighed and looked at me; I could see she was choosing her words carefully. 'You might be pleased to hear what I have to say,' she replied, smiling in an attempt to lighten the mood. 'I have to tell you that I've decided to go back to Germany to live with my parents because my father is getting old and isn't very well, so I'm afraid I shall be leaving.'

'Leaving? Ingrid you can't,' I replied. 'You're an excellent dental nurse and good nurses are very hard to find; I shall be terribly sorry to lose you. Aren't you happy here? Do you need more money?' I'm sure Spencer would be willing to increase your wages to keep you. He won't want you to leave either.'

'It's not about money and I've been happy here but my mother needs my support. I've very much enjoyed living in England but the time has now come for me to go back to Germany.'

'So your mind is made up?'

'It is, I'm afraid and now that I've made the decision I would like to leave as soon as possible but I'm prepared to stay on long enough to give Spencer time to find you another nurse.'

'It's a bitter blow, Ingrid, I shall miss you very much but you must do what you think is right. Have you told Spencer?'

'Yes, I told him earlier.'

'What did he say?'

'He just said he was sorry and that he'd start looking for someone else immediately.'

'It won't be easy. The girl he chose for me before you came was totally unsuitable – she had a phobia about needles, blood and dentures. Whatever made him think she would be any good I don't know – she couldn't have been more unsuitable and she only lasted a morning.'

'Perhaps he'll let you help him choose someone this time now that you're more established.'

'I very much doubt it. He thinks I'll choose someone for entirely the wrong reasons. He'd really like to find me someone of Beryl's age – someone to mother me and certainly no-one under thirty. He would have rejected you on the grounds that you were too young if there had been anyone else available.'

'That's utter rubbish,' interjected Spencer who suddenly appeared from nowhere. 'I knew that Ingrid would prove to be a good nurse as soon as I met her and I wasn't wrong was I? It is, however, a great shame that she wants to leave and I shall be very sorry to see her go but I understand and respect her reasons for going back to Germany.'

'It's going to be very difficult to replace her,' I responded gloomily.

'Well as it happens we might just be in luck. By sheer coincidence I was in the Red Lion last week and the landlord, Bill Cowan asked if I needed a dental nurse as he knew of someone who was looking for a job. Naturally I told him I didn't because at the time, I was unaware of Ingrid's plans but I phoned him this morning to see if she was still available and he said he thought she was. He said he'd get her to contact me as soon as possible.'

'She might not be any good at all,' I remarked unenthusiastically. 'Do you know anything about her? Has she any previous experience? How old is she? Does she live near here?'

'Slow down, Justin,' Spencer exclaimed. 'I don't know anything about her yet; we'll just have to wait and see.'

'Well please promise me you won't employ her unless she really is suitable. I still can't forget Sandra and what a complete disaster that was.'

'All right, all right, you don't need to keep on reminding me though I have to say I don't think you gave her a fair chance. I think you expected too much of her too soon bearing in mind that she had no previous experience of dental nursing.'

'Ingrid didn't either; the difference is she didn't pass out at the first sight of a needle or someone's denture.'

'Will you let Justin help you choose someone?' Ingrid asked. 'After all he's the one who will be working with her.'

'With all due respect I don't think Justin is sufficiently experienced to choose wisely; I think the selection process should be left to me,' Spencer replied. He began muttering to himself and it was clear that he felt slightly uncomfortable about refusing to allow me to play any part in choosing my nurse especially in view of fact that he had made a complete mess of it previously. He decided to change the subject.

'Haven't you got any patients?'

'I'm waiting for Mr Froy, who's always late.'

'Some patients are so infuriating,' he asserted and stormed off.

Mr Froy had an appointment for a small filling in an upper premolar. He rarely came on time and offered a variety of plausible excuses as to why he had been delayed ranging from the cat getting stuck up a tree to being detained by Jehovah's witnesses. The church clock struck the quarter hour which let me know he was already fifteen minutes late then I heard him running up the stairs pouring out abject apologies to Beryl for keeping me waiting. He was wearing his usual black leather jacket and winkle-picker shoes and his sleek, jet black hair positively glistened with hair cream.

'I'm so sorry I'm late, Mr Derwent. The taxi was late picking me up.'

He always came by taxi which surprised me somewhat because he was forever pleading poverty and I knew that he was claiming supplementary benefit which entitled him to free dental treatment. He also lived on a bus route which passed very close to the practice but claimed that the buses never ran on time so he didn't rely on them.

'You aren't going to do anything nasty to me today are you, Mr Derwent?' were his opening words.

'Of course not, Mr Froy,' I replied. 'I never do, do I?'

'I didn't like it one little bit when you took that tooth out for me last year.'

'I don't remember it being too bad; in fact it came out quite easily as I recall.'

'Well if that was easy, I dread to think what a difficult one would be like; it seemed quite a struggle to me. I don't suppose you've still got the tooth, have you?'

'I'm afraid not. It was over six months ago.'

'That's a shame. I thought you might have kept it.'

'Why on earth would I want to keep it, Mr Froy? Extracted teeth are a source of infection so they go straight into the clinical waste. Why do you ask?'

'I'm going to Ireland next week and I wanted to throw it in the Irish Sea. It's something of a tradition in our family; every one of my father's teeth finished up there.'

'I'm sorry but I haven't got it.'

'If I have another tooth out will you give it to me?'

'Hopefully you won't need any more extractions.'

'I hope so too but if I do, will you give it to me?'

'Yes, all right but now we need to get on with your filling. I'll just pop in an injection.'

'What, for a small filling?' he scoffed. 'That won't be necessary, Mr Derwent, I don't need an injection; I've got a very high pain threshold. Just get on with it; it'll be fine.'

I was pleased to hear this as I was anxious to make up some of the lost time. 'Are you sure, Mr Froy?'

'Absolutely.'

'Very well, then.' I picked up the drill and moved towards him but he wasn't ready to let me start yet. He was an avid follower of current affairs and had a habit of talking about the latest item of news which had captured his attention just as I was about to start his treatment.

'It's been an eventful week,' he commented, 'first Harold Wilson announces his resignation and then Princess Margaret and Lord Snowdon are getting a divorce.'

'Yes it has,' I agreed.

'Who do you think is likely to take over as Prime Minister?'

'I really don't know, Mr Froy. Will you open your mouth please?'

'I think Jim Callaghan will get the job. He'd be my choice anyway. Roy Jenkins would be my second choice but I think Callaghan will get it.'

'You may well be right, Mr Froy, now will you please open your mouth?'

'I'm surprised and disappointed to hear about Princess Margaret though. My view is that marriage is "till death us do part". I don't believe in divorce but that's just my view.'

I wasn't prepared to enter into discussion with him; I was very conscious of the fact that my next patient would be arriving very soon and I didn't want to keep her waiting. 'We need to get on with your filling, Mr Froy. I must ask you to stop talking and open your mouth.' I moved in closer and hovered over him with the drill.

'Yes of course, sorry, Mr Derwent, you must get on. I think things hadn't been right for some time though you know. Apparently there had been all sorts of funny goings on by both parties; drink and the rest amongst other things, so I've heard.'

'Is that so, Mr Froy? Will you please stop talking and let me get on with your filling?'

'I've also heard that Lord ….Snowdon …. is…..err….well, you know,' he whispered and winked at me.

'No, I don't know.'

He continued to whisper. 'Well it's only what I've heard, mind you; I don't know for sure and I can't swear that it's true but I've heard……. that he's a bit the other way, if you know what I mean. Though I'm not sure if there's any truth in it; it's only what I've heard.'

'That's fascinating, Mr Froy, but you must let me do your filling. Unless we get on, I shall be running late for the rest of the morning and all my patients will be kept waiting.' Ingrid picked up the saliva ejector and closed in on him from the other side and he finally fell silent and opened his mouth. As soon as the drill touched his tooth he jumped and drew his head away. 'That's mighty painful, Mr Derwent.'

'I haven't started yet. I think we're going to have to give you an injection.'

'No, I'm sorry. It just took me by surprise, that's all. Try again and I'll do my best to be brave.'

He closed his eyes and screwed up his face. Although his mouth was open, it was set in a contorted grimace and was barely wide enough for me see the tooth I needed to treat let alone drill it. 'You'll need to open wider than that, Mr Froy.'

His response was to part his lips by a further quarter of an inch. 'Still not wide enough I'm afraid.' His upper lip twitched and his jaw began to tremble. He managed to control it after a few moments then his mouth opened and closed several times like a goldfish's and finally came to rest with about an inch between his lips.

'I'm sorry, Mr Froy but I can't do your filling unless you open wider.' I put my fingers between his teeth and prised them apart until his mouth was wide enough for me to get the drill into position. I pressed the foot pedal to start the drill and immediately he clamped his lower teeth against it pushing the bur into his upper tooth. This caused the drill to stall and he let out an ear-splitting scream.

'Can't you be more gentle, Mr Derwent? That was really painful.'

'You drilled your own tooth by closing your mouth on the drill. You must keep wide open and it will be a lot less painful if you do.'

At that moment, the doorbell rang and I sighed because I knew it would be my next patient arriving and I was getting nowhere with Mr Froy.

'Can't you put me to sleep, Mr Derwent, then I won't feel anything?'

'I'm afraid I can't, Mr Froy but I could give you an injection.' I chuckled to myself to think that he was full of bravado before I started his treatment and now he was asking for a general anaesthetic. However, the realisation that I was getting later and later curtailed my moment of amusement.

'I don't really like injections,' he moaned. 'I hate the idea of having a needle stuck in me and I can't bear the feeling of numbness which seems to go on for ages afterwards. I don't know what to do. Can we try once more without an injection?'

'Very well but you must keep your mouth wide open.'

Slowly and reluctantly he opened his mouth. This time his eyes were wide open and rolling around as if he were intent on watching my every move. Ingrid slid a large saliva ejector between his teeth to try and prevent him from clamping his jaws together. I put the drill into position and as soon as I started it he let out another deafening screech and grabbed my hand to pull the drill away from his mouth. As he did so he bit so hard onto the saliva ejector that Ingrid was unable to pull it out of his mouth. When he finally released his grip, I was amazed to see that he had completely squashed the metal tube.

'I'm glad neither Ingrid nor I had our fingers in your mouth when you did that Mr Froy; you'd have bitten them clean off.'

'I'm sorry, Mr Derwent, I don't mean to be difficult but it was so painful. I don't know what the answer is.'

'I think the answer, Mr Froy, is for me to put a dressing in your tooth and arrange another appointment. When you come next time, I'll give you an injection before we start so you won't feel any pain. I know you don't like injections but there's no alternative.'

'I suppose you're right, Mr Derwent. I'm sorry for wasting your time.'

After Mr Froy left I tried desperately to make up the lost time but I didn't succeed and realised that my lunch break was going to be much shorter than planned. I was washing my hands after my last patient of the morning when Ingrid came into my surgery to tell me that lunch was going to be delayed even further.

'It's Reverend Jenkinson, Justin. He's still having trouble following his tooth extraction. He's in the waiting room. He didn't make an appointment but he said he couldn't stand the pain any longer so he just called in hoping you'd see him.'

'Oh dear, I've dressed the socket three times but it doesn't seem to be getting any better. All right, Ingrid, you'd better show him in.'

I was very sorry to hear that Reverend Jenkinson was still having trouble; he was a very likeable old man and not the sort to cause a fuss without good reason.

'Thank you so much for seeing me, Mr Derwent but I'm in absolute agony. I thought having a tooth out was supposed to stop toothache not cause it. It didn't hurt that much before you extracted it and now it's killing me.' In spite of his pain he was nevertheless able to raise a smile as he said it.

'Come and sit down, Reverend Jenkinson. It's obviously not the tooth that's hurting – the tooth's gone; you've got a dry socket.'

'What's that?'

'The socket is infected. A blood clot forms after a tooth is extracted but sometimes the blood clot is dislodged or destroyed leaving the surface of the bone exposed and it can then become infected.'

'I'm so sorry to keep troubling you but it's not getting any better.'

'It should be getting better by now. I've done everything recommended by the textbooks; I don't know why it isn't responding. Let me have a word with my colleague; he might have some bright ideas or some magic preparation we could try.'

Fortunately Spencer was still in his surgery and listened with interest when I told him that Reverend Jenkinson had developed a dry socket following the extraction of a lower molar five days ago.

'Poor old chap,' said Spencer sympathetically, 'he's been a patient of the practice for many years. He's a true Christian – always visiting the old and infirm or anyone in need of spiritual guidance. Apparently he reads the births, marriages and deaths columns in all the daily papers and writes to anyone he has been remotely acquainted with who has given birth or got married. If he reads that someone has died he always goes to their funeral; I reckon he's been to more funerals than I've had hot dinners. I'm not particularly religious but if anyone could convert me, he could.'

'Well he's got this dry socket and nothing I've done for him has been effective so far.'

'Dry sockets don't usually cause much trouble, Justin. What have you tried?' he asked superciliously.

Whenever I sought his advice he became extremely pompous and there was no doubt that he enjoyed adopting the role of consultant.

'I've tried irrigating it with saline, Eusol, and various other antiseptic solutions and I've packed it with gauze soaked in Whitehead's varnish but nothing seems to be doing any good.'

He shook his head as if pouring scorn on my choice of treatment even though this was the recommended course of action for dealing with dry sockets. 'I've never found any of those things to be very effective,' he sneered.

'So what do you use, Spencer?'

'Brown paste.'

'Brown paste? What's that?' I probed.

He went to his cupboard and pulled out an enormous glass jar which was half full of a paste like substance which was indeed brown.

'My father had it made up when he first went into practice, by a chemist in London. It lasted him throughout his entire practising career and I reckon it will see me through to retirement as well. It's wonderful stuff – you can use it for dry sockets, gum pockets, infected wisdom teeth; there's no end to its uses.'

'What's in it?' I queried.

'I haven't a clue,' Spencer admitted, as if its composition was immaterial. 'All I know is that it works.'

'It certainly smells strongly antiseptic,' I remarked, vainly attempting to identify some of its ingredients but I had to admit it smelt different from anything I had previously encountered.

'Stick some of that in his socket,' said Spencer with the utmost confidence. 'I'll guarantee it will stop his pain within twenty minutes and he won't have any more trouble.'

I looked at the mysterious mixture with suspicion and wondered if it was possible it could be so effective. If it was so

25

marvellous why wasn't it in any of the textbooks? I found it hard to believe that Spencer and his father were the only dentists to be privy to a universal panacea for minor oral infections but since everything I'd used so far had failed, there was no harm in giving it a try.

I went back to Reverend Jenkinson and tried to sound optimistic. 'I've got just the thing here – one of Mr Padginton's old fashioned remedies and one he swears by. It's something his father had made up apparently.'

'I knew his father well; he was a lovely man. My goodness it's got a very strong smell, Mr Derwent,' he remarked as I placed a large dollop of it into his infected socket. As I did so a small blob dropped on to his tongue and he recoiled. 'It doesn't taste too good, but I suppose the best medicines never do.'

'That's right. Anyway, let's see if it works. Try to eat and drink down the other side to avoid dislodging it.'

'I will, Mr Derwent and thank you. I hope it works because I'm conducting a wedding tomorrow. I'm retired really but they call me in from time to time if the usual vicar is ill or on holiday. I'm always very willing to help out. Forgive me for asking, Mr Derwent but do I detect a slight northern accent?'

'Yes, I was born and brought up in Sheffield.'

'Really? Whereabouts in Sheffield?'

'Heeley. Do you know it?'

'I certainly do, my first ministry was in Heeley – what a coincidence. That was a long, long time ago mind but isn't it a small world, Mr Derwent?'

'It certainly is, Reverend Jenkinson. Let me know how you get on with Mr Padginton's magic paste.'

'Yes I will and fancy you coming from Heeley. Well, well, what a surprise!'

CHAPTER FOUR

It was about six o'clock when I arrived home from the surgery that evening. Instinctively, I switched on the radio and flopped on to the sofa to unwind from the stresses of the day. It was a Friday and I was looking forward to a quiet weekend. I had no real plans but I thought I might go out with my camera as I was always on the lookout for that elusive stunning landscape photograph. I had come to realise, however, that success in that particular branch of photography was very dependent on the weather. The forecast for the weekend was warm and sunny so the prospects of a winning photograph were not great; stormy, unsettled weather would have been much more promising from a photographic point of view. These thoughts were running through my mind when the phone rang.

'Hello Justin, it's Sarah Hanson here. Do you remember me?'

'How could I forget? Last time we met you whacked me across the face.'

'I know, Justin, I'm so terribly, terribly sorry about that. I shouldn't have slapped your face; it was wrong of me. I've bitterly regretted it ever since. Are you still cross with me?'

She said it so sweetly and appealingly that even if I had still been annoyed with her, it would have been difficult to continue to be. It served as a reminder that when a woman turns on the charm, a man doesn't stand a chance.

'It was quite a long time ago now,' I remarked, trying to sound indifferent about it.

'It does seem a long time ago. I've been thinking about phoning you ever since it happened,' she continued. 'I'm really sorry for what I did. I wanted to apologise to you and I have been on the point of phoning several times but I always chickened out at the last minute because I thought you might be so annoyed, you wouldn't

27

want to see me ever again. I'm thoroughly ashamed of the way I behaved. Do you think you could ever forgive me?'

'As I said, it was a long time ago. It's more or less forgotten about.'

'Do you think we could meet to talk or are you seeing someone else now? I wouldn't want to intrude on your life if you are.'

'No, I'm not seeing anyone else. We can meet if you want to.'

'I really do Justin. In fact I'd love to meet up with you again. I realise now there was nothing serious between you and Annette. I know that, because I've seen her once or twice and we've talked about you. She very much wanted you to have a serious relationship with her but she admitted to me that you never led her on and you made it clear to her you only wanted friendship and nothing more.'

'It's a pity you didn't believe me when I told you. It would have saved a lot of unpleasantness.'

'I know it would and I was wrong to doubt you. I would like to try and make it up to you if you'll let me. I accept that you aren't looking for a deep relationship but can't we at least be friends?'

'Yes of course we can, Sarah, as long as you promise to keep your fists to yourself.' I said it jokingly and Sarah responded in the same vein.

'I promise faithfully not to lay a finger on you.'

'Well then, now that we've established the ground rules would you like me to take you out for a drink?'

'That would be lovely, Justin.'

'This evening?'

'Oh…err….well yes, all right, why not?'

'Are you sure?'

'Yes, I'd love to. My mother and I have something on over the weekend and we have an early start tomorrow morning but there's no real reason why that should stop me going out this evening.'

'I'll pick you up about quarter past eight. Will that be all right?'

'Yes, that'll be fine. Thank you, Justin; I'll see you later then.'

I went into the kitchen to find that I had very little food in the house. All I could rustle up was some baked beans and a couple of slices of stale bread which I toasted. Having taken the edge off my hunger, I sat for about ten minutes before taking a shower.

As I got in my car to go to meet Sarah, the church clock was striking eight. Since starting work with Spencer, the sound of the church clock had become very familiar to me. Its striking every quarter hour helped me to stay on time when treating patients. The fine old church was very close to the practice and had a magnificent tower, built around 1500, which dominated the landscape for miles around Luccombury. I didn't always hear the clock from my cottage; it seemed to depend on the wind direction but I could hear it very clearly that evening.

As I drove along, I was trying to decide how I felt about meeting Sarah again. I suppose, to be honest, I was pleased she phoned and I hadn't hesitated for a moment in offering to take her out for a drink, which must mean something. I had enjoyed her company previously and we got on well together until the business with Annette put an end to it. I liked to have female friends and Sarah was probably the sort of person who made a good friend. On other hand, I couldn't really cope if suddenly one of these friends wanted the association to become something more. At this stage of my life I wanted everything to remain as simple and straightforward as possible; I didn't feel ready for anything complicated. The big question for me was whether Sarah was happy to keep it that way, or did the fact that she had decided to phone me up mean she had other, more involved ideas about our future together. She had said she accepted I wasn't looking for a deep relationship, but life was beginning to show me that women didn't always mean what they say, or say what they mean.

Sarah was ready for me by her front door as I pulled into her drive. She looked very attractive in a white blouse and navy blue skirt. Her blond hair was shorter than when I last saw her and it suited her.

'Hello, Justin,' she called out, 'it's lovely to see you.'

'It's lovely to see you too, Sarah. You look well.'

I got out of my car and kissed her on the cheek. 'I thought we might drive down towards the coast and find a little pub somewhere along the way. There are some interesting places that I've not been in yet. How does that sound?'

'Absolutely fine,' Sarah replied, 'I really don't mind where we go. It will just be nice to talk.'

We drove for about eight miles and stopped at a little thatched pub called the Travellers' Rest. It wasn't very busy and we found a quiet table in a corner. I ordered some drinks and Sarah began the conversation. 'I'm truly sorry for what happened.'

'I know, Sarah, let's put it behind us now. It's a shame it happened and that it temporarily ended our friendship but it's all in the past and I'm prepared to forget about it.'

'I'm so glad, Justin, I was sure you would have found someone else by now, and that you would be in a steady relationship with someone special.'

'No, there's no-one special in my life. How about you?'

'I did meet someone and we went out together for a short time, but it didn't work out.'

'I'm sorry to hear that.'

'No, don't be. I could tell he wasn't really my type from the start. He had some very rowdy friends and they used to go out and get really drunk. I could accept him doing that once in a while but it happened a bit too often for my liking.'

'So you ended it?'

'Yes and I'm glad I did.'

We chatted for some considerable time, mostly about the Bankks Club and Ephraim with his Dinosaur skull. Finally Sarah asked if I minded taking her home because she and her mother had an early start next day. They had been invited to a wedding in Sussex and were driving up there, leaving home at 5.00 a.m.

'I'm sorry to end the evening early, Justin. I've had a lovely time,' said Sarah as we pulled up outside her house. 'I hope you'll come in for a quick cup of coffee, though, and I'd like you to meet my mother.'

'I don't want to keep you up. You must be anxious to get to bed.'

'No, really, please come in just for a short time.'

'All right, then, as long as you're sure and throw me out when you want to go to bed.'

As soon as Sarah opened the front door, we were met by a furry welcoming committee. 'This is Winnie,' said Sarah introducing me to a little, black, smooth-haired mongrel, 'and this is Tigger. Say hello to Justin, girls.'

Tigger was much bigger and mostly border collie. Both dogs were very friendly, though it was clear that Tigger was much more dominant than Winnie and pushed her smaller companion out of the way to gain Sarah's affection. They were both delighted to see Sarah come home.

'Come and meet my mother.'

Sarah led me into the sitting room, where a frail and very pale looking, well-dressed lady in her sixties was watching television. She immediately turned it off as we entered.

'Mother, this is Justin. Justin, meet my mother.'

'How do you do, Mrs Hanson,' I said, shaking her hand.

'Sit down, Justin and I'll go and make some coffee. Would you like some, mother?'

'No thank you, dear, I had some earlier. If I have any more I won't be able to sleep.'

The dogs were quite intrigued by their new visitor and wouldn't leave me alone. Tigger kept licking my hand and demanding that I keep on stroking her. Winnie brushed back and forth against my legs before finally jumping up on to my lap.

'That's most unusual,' Sarah's mother remarked, 'Winnie is usually very wary of strangers, particularly men, but she obviously likes you, Justin. Look at this, Sarah,' she called out as Sarah came through from the kitchen with two mugs of coffee. 'The dogs have taken to Justin immediately.'

'Yes that is unusual,' Sarah agreed. 'They don't meet many men in the house and they're usually very shy with them.'

'You obviously have a way with animals, Justin,' said Sarah's mother, 'do you have any pets of your own?'

'No I don't. In fact, the only pet I've ever owned was a budgerigar when I was about ten. I love animals but it wasn't possible to have one whilst I was a student and it would still be difficult, being at work all day. I'd like a dog but I wouldn't want to leave it on its own for long periods; I don't think it would be fair on the dog.'

'No, you're right. Dogs love you to be with them – they can get quite distressed if they're left on their own too long. In fact, I'm a bit worried about tomorrow. We'll be leaving very early tomorrow morning to get to this wedding and it'll be late when we get back. Sometimes, one of the neighbours will pop in to feed the dogs and let them have a run on the rare occasions that we do go out for the day but she's away this week. I almost felt like saying we couldn't go to the wedding but I really feel that we have to go. It's the daughter of a special friend who's getting married.' She paused for a few moments. 'I don't suppose you'd be prepared to look in on them, Justin, would you?'

Sarah rapidly intervened. 'Mother you can't expect Justin to do that. He probably has other plans for tomorrow.'

'I honestly don't mind. I haven't any plans for tomorrow. I can look in on them and feed them if you like.'

'Are you sure, Justin?' said Sarah. 'That really is very kind of you. Mother had no right to ask you. I feel very embarrassed that she should put you on the spot like that within a few minutes of meeting you.'

'That's all right. I'm more than happy to help – they are such lovely dogs. What would you like me to do?'

I drank my coffee and Sarah showed me where the dogs' leads, food and feeding bowls were kept and she gave me a set of keys for the house.

'I'll pop in around lunchtime,' I promised, as Sarah led me back to my car. 'Have a lovely day tomorrow and don't worry about the dogs – I'll look after them.'

'Justin, it is so very kind of you, thank you so much. I've had a lovely time tonight. I hope we will be able to see each other again.'

She took hold of my hand and kissed me quickly on the lips. It was quite affectionate but restrained. I squeezed her hand and lightly touched her shoulder to let her know that her kiss was not unwelcome.

CHAPTER FIVE

I drove to Sarah's house at about twelve-thirty. The sun was shining and I thought that if the weather was like this in Sussex, it would be a lovely day for the wedding. It seemed strange to be going into someone else's house and it crossed my mind that if any of the neighbours could see me, they might think I was an intruder. I certainly hoped that the police would not turn up, demanding to know what I was up to. No doubt I would be able to prove my innocence eventually but I could well do without the hassle. Fortunately that didn't happen and I was able to unlock the door and go into the house without any problem.

I was slightly wary of the dogs. They had been fine with me whilst Sarah and her mother were present, but how would they feel when I entered the house unaccompanied? Would they see me as a burglar and adopt the role of guard dogs, protecting their territory? Surely Sarah and her mother would not have asked me to go in and feed them if there had been any danger that the dogs might become aggressive. They looked friendly enough as they came out into the hall wagging their tails. I was sure they were harmless and they let me stroke them, but understandably, they did seem to be slightly cautious though perhaps it was just my imagination.

Sarah had asked me to feed them and let them run out into the garden for a while. She hadn't said in which order. Should I feed them first or let them out first? I wasn't really sure – perhaps it didn't matter. I decided the best thing to do would be to let them out and whilst they were running around outside, I would fill their food bowls so that when they came back, the food would be on the floor ready for them to eat. After they had eaten, I would let them out once more for a while so they could get some fresh air before being shut in again. After all, it would be quite a long time before Sarah and her mother got back home.

I thought it was a reasonable plan so I opened the back door and tried to persuade them to venture forth into the garden. However, they clearly did not wish to go out at that moment. They both sat down on the kitchen floor looking at me demandingly. I went outside and called to them to join me, but they didn't respond. If they had been able to speak, they couldn't have told me any more clearly that they weren't going to do anything until they'd been fed.

I opened the tins of dog food and spooned it into their bowls. My intention was to place the bowls on the floor some feet away from them and then give the command for them to go over and eat. Tigger, however, had other ideas and she leapt at the bowl, knocking it clean out of my hand. The food went all over the floor and Tigger pounced on it gulping it down as if she hadn't eaten anything for six months. In an instant she had cleaned up every scrap, not just from the bowl but also from the floor around it. Winnie, on the other hand, was far better mannered. I put her bowl down and she walked demurely towards it with a level of decorum, which belied her lack of pedigree. But sadly for her, Tigger lunged across knocking the little dog out of the way and then she began wolfing down Winnie's food.

I couldn't stand back and watch this happen so I tried to intervene by pushing Tigger away. Her response was to growl and snap at my hand, drawing blood from my left thumb. I tried again to recover Winnie's bowl. This time Tigger turned and snarled at me in an alarmingly menacing way. I was forced to retreat as Tigger, growling and exposing her huge canine teeth, advanced towards me. She was intent on making sure I was far enough away from the bowl to allow her to continue to devour Winnie's food without further interference from me. I knew little about dogs, but I had heard or read that it is fatal to let a dog sense that you are afraid of it – apparently they can smell the fear. All I can say is that the scent of fear would have been very powerful at that moment and my first impulse was to run out of the kitchen into the garden and shut the door behind me. It then crossed my mind that the worst thing you can do, according to what I had heard and read, when faced with a vicious dog, is to try and run away from it. I didn't run, probably because fear had me rooted to the spot, but fortunately for me, once Tigger was certain I was far enough away from the food to be ineffective in keeping her from it, she turned away from me and pounced upon the remaining meat, whilst poor little Winnie just stood back and watched. I did the same from the other side of the room.

I had no choice but to allow Tigger to finish up the last morsel of Winnie's dinner and then lick the bowl clean. Once she had accomplished this, her temperament reverted back to that of a pussycat.

I was concerned that Winnie hadn't had the opportunity to eat anything but there didn't seem to be anything I could do about it. If I produced more food, undoubtedly Tigger would make sure she got hold of it and I couldn't face being savaged by her a second time. My thumb was quite painful and still bleeding. I picked up the bowls and washed them under the tap. Tigger was still licking the kitchen floor in case there might be a taste of something still there but the ferocity had gone out of her. I put the bowls away and invited the dogs to go out into the garden; an invitation they readily accepted.

I let them play in the garden for about twenty minutes and eventually they came back into the kitchen of their own accord, which I took as an indication that they had had enough fresh air. I gave them a stroke, made sure they had plenty of water and then I let myself out, carefully locking the door behind me.

CHAPTER SIX

I was half expecting Sarah to phone when she and her mother got back. I don't know why, but I just had a feeling she might. However, when it got to midnight and she still hadn't contacted me I decided she probably wouldn't now, so I went to bed. My head just touched the pillow when the phone rang. I knew it would be her.

'I'm sorry to phone you so late, Justin, but we've only just got back. We had a terrible journey, the traffic was very heavy and there were three lots of road works.'

'You must both be very tired. It's been a very long day for you.'

'We are a bit tired but I wanted to speak to you and thank you for looking after the dogs. They seem fine. I think they slept most of the time. How did you get on?'

'I've just got back from accident and emergency having had my thumb sewn back on.'

'Oh my God, Justin, poor you, whatever happened? I'll come over right away and look after you.'

'No, no, Sarah, I'm only joking. I didn't really have to go to hospital.'

'Then why on earth did you say it? Please don't joke like that, my heart turned over. Have you hurt your thumb?'

'Tigger had a go at me. She bit my thumb and made it bleed but it isn't too bad. She gulped her food down and then decided to push Winnie out of the way and steal hers. When I tried to intervene she bit me.'

'Oh, Justin, I'm so sorry. I should have warned you that she can get a bit aggressive when there's food at stake. She knows mother and I won't stand for it, so she doesn't try to do it when we feed them, but I suppose she thought she could take advantage of you. She's as good as gold and gentle as a lamb, except when it comes to food. I think it's because she had a poor start in life. She was one of eight puppies and the owner didn't feed them properly; he just used to throw food down and they had to fight for it in order to survive. The RSPCA rescued the puppies and that's how we came get Tigger.'

'She certainly got aggressive. After biting my thumb she turned and started to advance towards me looking as if she would tear me to pieces; I was quite scared of her.'

'I'm so sorry, Justin. I'm sure she wouldn't really have hurt you.'

Sarah sounded sorry, but I could tell she was trying not to laugh at the same time.

'It isn't funny you know Sarah.'

'I know it isn't, Justin, and I don't mean to laugh. It's just the thought of you being frightened of Tigger, who has the sweetest nature you could wish for in a dog.'

'She didn't look all that sweet to me this afternoon. If you'd seen the way she bared her teeth at me – it was terrifying.'

'She honestly wouldn't have attacked you viciously. She behaved as she did so that she could get her own way, but it was all surface show. She's never attacked anyone in her life; she wouldn't – it's not in her nature. If you'd stood up to her she would have backed down. I am truly grateful to you, though, for going in to feed them. Please let me come over and look at your thumb. Does it need bandaging?'

'No, it'll be all right. I don't want you to come over tonight. You've had a very long day and you need to get some rest. My thumb's fine, really. You ought to give Winnie some food, though, because she didn't manage to get a single mouthful earlier on.'

'I'll see that she gets something. Are you really sure you don't want me to come over and look after you?'

'I'm really sure, Sarah, but thank you for offering.'

'When can I see you again, Justin?' It would be lovely to go out together when I didn't have to get up so early next morning. Can I see you tomorrow, or I should say later today as it's after midnight?'

'I'm sorry, but I'm tied up tomorrow. I'm ... err...going to meet an old university friend who's in the area this weekend. I'll give you a ring during the week.'

'That's a shame, but it will be nice for you to meet your friend. Have you met up since leaving university?'

'Err....no.'

'Then you'll no doubt have a lot to talk about. I'll wait for you to contact me then, Justin, but don't leave it too long will you? And thank you once again for looking after the dogs. Good night and sleep well.'

'Good night, Sarah.'

I put down the phone and went back to bed but I it was a long time before I was able to get to sleep – I was too preoccupied with thinking about Sarah. She was a lovely girl and I liked her very much, but I suppose alarm bells were beginning to ring. Before yesterday, I hadn't seen or heard from her for several months. She phoned and I took her out for a drink – no harm in that – but why did she feel it was necessary to phone tonight, after midnight? Couldn't it have waited until tomorrow? It was very kind of her to offer to come over and tend to my injured thumb, but to offer to do so at that time of night, after a long tiring day, was going beyond the call of duty. She also wanted to see me again tomorrow. I wasn't proud of myself for lying to her about meeting a university friend but I just felt I needed a bit of breathing space and some time to think. I was worried that Sarah was suddenly trying to move things along much too quickly, though perhaps I was unduly hasty and over cautious in thinking that. Perhaps I was worrying unnecessarily and doing her an injustice.

The decision I reached finally was that I definitely wanted to go on seeing Sarah but it was vital for us to take things slowly and one step at a time. I could easily become very claustrophobic where women were concerned. My experience with Annette was still very fresh in my mind and to some extent I blamed myself for allowing it to get out of hand. The truth was that I had relatively little experience of the opposite sex and I had never previously been involved in a truly serious relationship. I had been out with girls whilst I was at university but it was always very casual and uninvolved and I suppose I felt comfortable with that. I didn't really feel ready for anything more at this stage of my life. Would I ever feel ready for anything more? I couldn't say. Presumably I would meet someone one day who would change my feelings on the matter. It probably wouldn't happen overnight – it would be a gradual process and maybe Sarah was that person. I didn't know. Only time would tell. In the meantime I hoped I would be able to enjoy her company, and for her to enjoy mine, without allowing things to spiral out of control.

CHAPTER SEVEN

'Good morning, Spencer.' I called out, as I passed the open door of his surgery.

'Oh, yes, good morning, Justin.'

It was a hesitant and pensive reply. He was deep in thought about something. I decided not to disturb him and went straight into the office where Beryl was filing some record cards.

'Spencer has something on his mind this morning,' she remarked. 'I came in early and he was deeply engrossed in something at his desk, and hardly spoke to me. I took him a cup of coffee, but I couldn't get any conversation out of him.'

'It wasn't his weight chart, was it?'

'No, I don't think so. He only gets that out before he goes away on holiday and I don't think he's planning on going anywhere at the moment. I really don't know what's occupying his thoughts.'

'I'm sure we'll find out soon enough.'

'What on earth have you done to your thumb, Justin?' she exclaimed suddenly, as she noticed it was bandaged up.

'I got bitten by a dog.'

'My goodness, how did that happen?'

I related the incident with Tigger and Beryl looked horrified.

'People who own dogs really annoy me. They always say, "it won't hurt you" when it's blatantly obvious to everyone else that the blooming thing is intent on taking a chunk out of your leg. They don't seem to realise that dogs don't look upon their owners and strangers in the same way.'

'Apparently I was too soft with the dog. I should have shown it who was boss.'

'It's easy to say that, but when you're faced with a ferocious beast bearing down on you it's very difficult to put theory into practice. Anyway, how on earth are you going to work with your thumb bandaged up like that?'

'I was going to take off the bandage and get Ingrid to put on a plaster. I could wear some rubber gloves to keep the plaster in place. It isn't too bad really.'

'Did you go to the hospital with it?'

'No, I didn't think it was bad enough for that.'

'Have you had a tetanus injection?' she asked, suddenly looking very concerned.

'No I shouldn't think I need one.'

'You ought to have one – you certainly don't want tetanus. You must have had an injection at some time in the past, haven't you?'

'I can't recall ever having one.'

'Then you really ought to get one, not just for this, but you never know when you might injure yourself on a rusty nail or cut yourself gardening. I do think you should go to the doctor or the hospital, just to be on the safe side.'

'I can't go today; I'm fully booked all day.'

'Well go to the hospital after work; they'll do it for you.'

'I don't know – I'll think about it. Ah, here comes Ingrid, I'll get her to change this bandage for a plaster.'

I went through the whole doggy incident with Ingrid who thought it was highly amusing.

'I don't know why anyone should think it funny.' I said grumpily, 'even Sarah started laughing when I told her what had happened.'

'I'm sorry, Justin. It's one of those situations that's funny to everyone except the person attacked by the dog.'

Ingrid removed the bandage and looked at the wound. 'It's only a little scratch; you can hardly call it a bite. I expected to see your thumb hanging off – bitten halfway through.'

'Thanks very much. It bled quite profusely at the time.'

'I'll put a plaster on it but I really don't think it's anything to worry about.'

'You should still get a tetanus jab though,' added Beryl. 'Apparently it's usually a little scratch – one that almost goes unnoticed, that lets in the infection. You often read about it.'

'I suppose you're right, Beryl, I'll think about going for a jab after work.'

With typical German detachment, Ingrid scoffed, 'It's nothing; I don't know why you're getting concerned about it. You English can be very wimpy at times.'

I found that a pair of surgical rubber gloves went over the plaster quite well but as I wasn't used to wearing gloves, I thought they might feel somewhat awkward. I would probably get used to them – after all, surgeons wear them all the time when operating. I was checking them out with some instruments when Spencer came through the door looking very excited. I thought he might wonder why I was wearing gloves and ask me. However, he had far more important things on his mind.

'You'll be delighted to know that I've found you a new nurse, Justin. The girl Bill Cowan told me about telephoned me and came to see me over the weekend.'

'That was quick, Spencer; it sounds too good to be true,' I responded coolly. 'Don't tell me; you managed to convince her that she couldn't afford to live on her old-age pension alone and you persuaded her to come out of retirement to help us out?'

'You can be really cynical at times, Justin. In fact she's young, blonde, attractive, quite vivacious, and she's a qualified dental nurse with considerable experience and her name's Wendy. I think you'll be very pleasantly surprised.'

'Young? I don't believe it. As I said, she sounds too good to be true. There must be a catch somewhere.'

'There's no catch. I think it's a stroke of good fortune that she happened to be available just at the right time. In fact her youth is the only possible thing I might not be entirely happy about; in every other respect she seems perfect.'

'When can she start?' asked Ingrid who appeared to share my scepticism though maybe she felt slightly hurt to think she could be replaced quite so quickly and easily.

'She's available immediately,' Spencer enthused.

'In that case,' said Ingrid, 'I'll leave at the end of the week if that's all right with you.'

'It has to be your decision, my dear,' Spencer proclaimed, suddenly aware that he might be hurting Ingrid's feelings. 'Please don't feel you are being pushed out but you did say you wanted to leave as soon as possible.'

'Yes I did and it would suit me to leave at the end of the week as I want to get back to Germany as soon as possible.'

'We must arrange a leaving party for you on Friday evening,' Spencer declared. 'I'm determined to give you a good send off.'

'Please don't,' Ingrid pleaded. 'I hate goodbyes and leaving parties; I would much rather just leave quietly.'

'You can't do that,' Spencer protested. 'You've been a great asset to the practice and I want to thank you properly for all you've done. I'm sure Justin will feel the same.'

'I really don't want it, Spencer; please believe me.'

Spencer looked quite hurt. He loved all parties whatever their motivation and found it hard to understand how anyone could have different views. 'If you're absolutely sure then I must respect your wishes. You will keep in touch with us won't you?'

'I promise I'll write to you and I intend visiting England from time to time; when I do, I shall come and see you.'

'We shall look forward to that won't we, Justin?'

'Most definitely. I'm still very upset that you're leaving, Ingrid. If the new girl turns out to be half as good as you I shall have nothing to complain about.'

'Now there's something else I want to talk about,' Spencer continued. 'We obviously have a problem getting patients like Lady Gascoyne-Fairley upstairs and I think I've come up with a way round it.' He sounded as if he had given the matter a considerable amount of thought and I felt sure he was about to come out with something very profound.

'Really, Spencer, what's that, a stair-lift?'

'No, no, more radical than that and a much better solution. We'll move the entire practice downstairs. The waiting room will become my new surgery. It's directly below my present surgery and is exactly the same size and shape, so that will work well. The only drawback from my point of view is that I will have to give up my indoor workshop, which is in the back room downstairs. That will become the new waiting room, and our sitting room will become your surgery. The downstairs kitchen will be the staff room, and the room that Daphne uses as her office will be the office for the practice. It will be a much better arrangement than at present because it means that the practice will be completely separate from our living accommodation. We will effectively be creating a flat upstairs and Daphne and I will live over the shop, so to speak.'

'It's going to be a major upheaval isn't it, Spencer?'

'I don't think it will be too bad – we can do it in stages. How do you feel about moving your surgery into our sitting room?'

'It's a great idea. It's much more spacious than the room I'm in at present and it's at the front of the house so, like you, I'll be able to see who's arriving.'

'I thought you might be pleased. Okay, the first job is to clear my workshop and turn it into the new waiting room. Having done that, I'll move my surgery downstairs into the old waiting room. We can move you downstairs later on to complete the move.'

'Does this mean you'll be buying new equipment for your surgery?'

'I'm seriously looking into it, Justin. I certainly think the time has come to move the practice forward to show all our patients that we are progressive and abreast of all the latest innovative developments in dentistry. I know we have a lot of old patients who don't really worry about these things but I notice that quite a lot of young families are moving into the area and we want to be sure that ours is the practice to attract them. In addition, and perhaps even more important, we have to think about the friends and contacts of the likes of Lady Gascoyne-Fairley. Many of these people go to London – Harley Street mostly, thinking that's where they'll get the best dental treatment. We have to show them that they can get treatment every bit as good, here in rural Dorset. They will, of course, be comparing our practice with the London practices so we have to make sure they'll be impressed with what they see.'

'How long is the move going to take?'

'I don't think we can afford to let it take too long. I shall be seeing a lot of Lady Gascoyne-Fairley and I want to be able to treat her downstairs as soon as possible. I'm thinking weeks, rather than months. It will obviously take some time to move you and the office downstairs, but I want to get my surgery sorted out very quickly. I shall have my workshop cleared out by the weekend and it will need smartening up a bit. I was hoping you might be prepared to give up some of your spare time to help put a lick of paint on the walls. Once we have that up and running as the waiting room, I can move my surgery downstairs. I might have to get the dental supply company's engineer to help me move the equipment, though hopefully, it won't be necessary.'

'You probably will need some help, Spencer. You can't possibly do it all yourself. But if you buy new equipment, the dental company will install it for you.'

'Yes, I suppose they will. Anyway that's a little way off yet. First we need to get the new waiting room ready.'

My immediate thought was that 'smartening up a bit' was something of an understatement with regards to Spencer's workshop. I didn't go in there very often, but my memory of it was that the walls were absolutely filthy. As it had been used as a workshop in connection with his vintage cars for many years, it had never really been decorated. Some of the plaster was cracked and falling off the walls and ceiling, but the most striking feature was that the entire floor was impregnated with oil and grease, and there was an overpowering reek of engine oil. It smelt more like the premises of a motor engineer than a room in a house, and I had grave doubts that it would be possible to eradicate the odour. The walls, which were to receive a euphemistic 'lick of paint', were covered in dust and grime.

'I think it's a very good idea to move the practice downstairs,' I agreed. 'We do have a lot of elderly patients and it will make life very much easier. I also think that re-equipping your surgery will do a lot to improve the image of the practice.'

Spencer made no comment so I continued. 'As far as decorating is concerned, I'm more than happy to help – just tell me what you want me to do.'

'Thanks, Justin. If you could spare some time at the weekend I'd be really grateful.'

Throughout the day I kept thinking about Spencer's plans to re-organise the practice. In a way, it seemed out of character, as normally he was strongly opposed to any sort of change. I couldn't believe he was thinking of discarding all the equipment that his father had installed some thirty years previously. He had always expressed much disdain for everything modern and maintained that his equipment was far better made and would outlast anything you could buy today. Perhaps the episode with Lady Gascoyne-Fairley had set him thinking and made him realise at last, that in order to keep up appearances he would have to move forward from the past. Modern equipment, after all, did have many advanced features, which, in the end, made the practice of dentistry more efficient and in many ways easier. Perhaps Spencer was beginning to recognise that.

I certainly liked the idea of moving my surgery from a relatively small back room upstairs to a lovely, spacious, downstairs room at the front of the house but the thought crossed my mind that if Spencer were to spend what would be quite a considerable sum of money on his surgery, he wouldn't be prepared to spend anything much on mine. There would be no possibility of new equipment for me. The equipment in my surgery was only slightly less antiquated than Spencer's, and by comparison, would look even worse if Spencer had a super new look to his. The thought depressed me somewhat. I wasn't a partner in the practice – I was only his associate but I had no wish to be considered the poor relation.

I wondered exactly how much it would cost to re-equip a dental surgery. I really hadn't much idea but I decided to find out. I was thinking that perhaps I could buy some new equipment; I could probably get a loan or buy it on hire purchase – there seemed to be lots of finance companies desperate to lend money to dentists if the advertisements in the monthly dental magazines were anything to go by.

It would be an unusual step for an associate to take, as normally the practice owner is responsible for providing the surgery for his associate, but I appreciated that Spencer probably wouldn't be able to afford to buy new equipment for both surgeries. Although I wasn't a partner in the practice, I felt settled there and I couldn't really see myself moving, so what did it matter? I felt sure that Spencer would not have any objections to the idea. After all, it would help to improve the overall image of the practice so he would benefit as well. I began to feel quite excited at the prospect of having some of the latest and most modern equipment and couldn't wait to make enquiries about obtaining some. I decided not to mention it to Spencer at this stage until I had done some costing to see whether or not my plan was viable.

CHAPTER EIGHT

When I arrived home after work I was still thinking about the prospect of having a brand new, state-of-the-art surgery in what was, at present, Spencer's spacious sitting room. It could be very impressive indeed and would make treating patients so much more enjoyable. For a while, my thoughts kept drifting as I tried to visualise how I would arrange things, then suddenly, I remembered that I had more or less decided to follow Beryl's advice to go for a tetanus injection, so thoughts of reconfiguring the practice would have to be put on hold. I would have to drive to Dorchester hospital, which would take me a little over half an hour, and before I set off I thought I would grab a bite to eat. I went to the larder to see if I had anything in the house.

As often seemed to happen whenever I started to do something, I was interrupted by the phone. I immediately thought that it would be Sarah.

'Hello, Justin. It's Richard Darcy here.'

'Hello, Richard. How are you?'

'Not too bad now but I felt a bit funny over the weekend. I felt slightly dizzy and a little bit hot, I really don't know what the trouble was, but I feel better today.'

'That's good. What are you up to?'

'Not a lot really. Things have been very quiet for the past couple of weeks; there didn't seem to be much about.'

I knew from experience that when he said there hadn't been much about, he meant he hadn't been very successful in picking up women.

'Where have you been looking?' I enquired, expecting a comprehensive list of all the nightclub and pubs in the area.

'The usual haunts but they've been very quiet. I heard today, though, of a new wine bar that has opened recently in Westport. I know someone who tried it about ten days ago and he didn't think it was all that good, but my friend John went there last Thursday and he said it looked promising, so the jury is still out at present. I thought I might look in there this evening and I wondered if you would like to come with me.'

'I might be able to, later on, Richard, but I'm just setting off to go to the hospital to get a tetanus injection. I don't know how long I shall be there.'

'Why on earth are you going for a tetanus injection?'

'I got bitten by a dog over the weekend and I thought I ought to have a jab, to be on the safe side.'

'Bitten by a dog? Blimey, that's terrible. Whose dog was it? Are you suing the owner?'

'No, I'm not suing; it was a friend's dog.'

'What kind of a friend is that, who let's their dog bite you?'

'It's a girl I've been out with a couple of times, called Sarah Hanson, do you know her?'

'I've met her. She's a nice looking girl. I met her about three months ago. I can't remember where it was now. I bought her a drink and asked for her telephone number but she was evasive and I didn't manage to get it. I think someone else came in at that point, someone she knew and she started talking to them, so I didn't get another chance. How did you manage to get bitten? Don't tell me. You were trying it on with Sarah and the dog came to her rescue?'

'No. Nothing like that. She and her mother went away for the weekend and they asked me to go in to feed the dogs. One of them got a bit greedy and attacked me when I tried to stop it eating the other dog's food as well as its own.'

My explanation prompted Richard to launch into his courtroom role as Counsel for the Prosecution.

'Members of the jury, you are being asked by the defendant to believe this ludicrous account of events, whereby he claims he was bitten whilst trying to feed two dogs. I put it to you that a far more likely scenario is that this loyal and faithful animal was desperately trying to defend its owner against the unwelcome advances of a sex-craved young dentist.'

'Sarah wasn't there. I told you she and her mother went to a wedding and I was asked to go in to look after the dogs.'

'It's terrible that you were bitten. That in itself is bad enough but are you suggesting you could go on to contract some horrible disease as a result, unless you get an injection to prevent it?'

'It isn't very likely but it could happen and it isn't worth taking the risk.'

'Good God, no. I'd be wetting myself if I thought I might contract something like that. Why didn't you get a tetanus injection straightaway?'

'I didn't really think about it. One of the nurses at work suggested I ought to get a jab. I don't think I've ever had one before and it's best to be protected because you can get tetanus quite easily, if you cut yourself whilst gardening, for example. You're particularly at risk if you get a cut contaminated by soil.'

'Oh my God, are you? Can you get tetanus that easily?'

'Yes you can. I don't think it's very common; but it can happen.'

'Oh dear, oh dear. That's terrible. I injured myself whilst I was pruning some roses over the weekend; I'm not likely to get it from that am I? I don't think I've ever had a tetanus jab.'

'It's not likely but theoretically it's possible.'

'So I might do? You can't be sure? Oh my God, it makes you think that it's best not to do any gardening – it's just not worth the risk.'

'It isn't just gardening. You can get it from any wound that punctures the skin if you get dirt in it.'

'Can you really? That's scary. You're bound to cut yourself occasionally however careful you are. You've got me very worried now. If I think about it, I must have cut myself three or four times in the past six months. I could have got tetanus from any of these injuries.'

'You'd have known about it by now, the symptoms start about a week after you get infected.'

'What are the symptoms?'

'Well from what I can remember from my pathology studies you start off with stiffness of the jaw and difficulty swallowing. You probably also have a high temperature and later you find you can't open your mouth.'

'Lockjaw?'

'Exactly. You get spasm of the facial muscles, which produces a characteristic expression with a fixed smile and elevated eyebrows known as risus sardonicus.'

'Hell's bells, that's horrendous; it sounds likes something out of a horror movie.'

'Then you get rigidity or spasm of the abdominal, neck and back muscles and the slightest noise or movement can trigger off painful generalised muscle spasms.'

'Stop, stop I can't bear to hear any more.'

Richard was sounding quite panic stricken now but I hadn't finished. 'The chest may become rigid, interfering with breathing, you will be sweating profusely and then you'll probably go into a coma. Death will follow soon after.'

'Oh my God, my God. I told you I felt hot at the weekend, I've got it, haven't I?'

'Calm down, it's most unlikely. It's also unlikely that I'll get it from the dog bite, but I'm not taking any chances.'

'It might be unlikely but you can't be sure. It would be terrible if I got it, Justin. I'm terrified of getting something like that. You don't really think I've got it do you? Do you think feeling hot at the weekend was a sign I've got it?'

'This was supposed to be about me getting tetanus from a dog bite, Richard. Now it seems to be all about you.'

'I know but it would be terrible if I got it.'

'Well I wouldn't be too happy if I got it, that's why I'm going for a jab.'

I was aware of a curious sound, which could best be described as high-pitched groaning at the other end of the phone. Finally, Richard spoke.

'I'd better come to the hospital with you and get a jab myself. Will you pick me up?' He sounded breathless and slightly hysterical.

'Yes, if you're sure you want to come. I'll pick you up in about half an hour.'

I made a cup of tea and briefly sat down to eat a hastily made cheese and tomato sandwich before setting out to pick up Richard. As I locked my front door, my landlord, Ephraim Trivett, called out to me. He was wearing the same grey cap he always wore and the same checked shirt he had on last week and the week before. Either he had several shirts all the same or he wore the same one continuously for weeks on end. I was inclined to think it was the latter. His black mongrel dog, Nellie, was by his side.

'Evenin', Justin. How 'ee be?'

'Not too bad, thanks Ephraim.'

'Is 'ee off out?'

'Yes, as a matter of fact I'm heading for Dorchester hospital.'

'Ah, na that cud be right 'andy.'

'In what way, Ephraim?'

'I 'as there a dozen young pigeons.' He pointed to a large carrying basket by the side of his shed. I could see that it contained several birds.

'I was takin' 'em off to release 'em. Not too far away like. I jus' wanted to start trainin' 'em up. Gettin' 'em ready for proper races. If 'ee be goon' to Dorchester, 'ee could tak em wi' 'ee and let 'em out there. If 'ee don't mind that is. Save me goin' out. I can just sit 'ere an' wait fer 'em to come back. Does 'ee mind?'

'No, I don't mind, it's just that the basket is quite big and my car is very small. It won't fit into my boot.'

'It'll fit on passenger seat.'

'Yes I suppose it will.' I was mindful of the fact that I would be picking up Richard and the only way I would be able to get him and the pigeons in my two-seater sports car would be to put the basket on his lap. I didn't think he would be keen on that idea but I wanted to help Ephraim and I liked his pigeons.

'Okay, Ephraim bring the basket over.'

The basket fitted onto the passenger seat without any problem and I drove to Richard Darcy's house. I had the hood folded down on my car as it was a pleasant evening and I could hear the music emanating from Richard's house from fifty yards away. Every time I had gone to visit him he was playing classical music at tremendous volume and I was surprised his neighbours were so tolerant. I parked on the road outside and rang his doorbell. He opened the door almost immediately.

'I'll just turn this down,' he began. He looked distinctly worried and his demeanour was even more twitchy than usual. 'You don't think I've got tetanus do you Justin? I've got all the symptoms. I told you I was hot and my face and jaw feel a bit stiff. My stomach muscles feel a bit tight as well. I haven't been able to eat a thing this evening; I just don't feel like it. Is loss of appetite a symptom as well?'

'You don't feel like eating because you've got yourself all worked up and that's probably why your stomach muscles feel tight.'

'But it would be terrible if I got tetanus.'

'It would be terrible if any of us got tetanus that's why we're going to the hospital. Now come on, turn off the music and let's go.'

Richard went through his usual routine of checking that every plug in the house was removed from the socket. After checking upstairs, he did three circuits of his sitting room on hands and knees ensuring that all plugs had been removed and the switches on the sockets were set to the off position. He then went into the kitchen to check the plugs and to make sure the fridge door was closed and the cooker turned off. Having satisfied himself that everything was safe, he instructed me to leave the house and he locked the door behind him pushing hard against it at least six times in order to certify that it was properly locked. Finally we were ready to depart.

'Can you put the hood up?' he asked, as soon as he set eyes on my car parked a few yards down the road. 'I might catch cold with the draught.'

'That'll be the least of your worries if you've got tetanus.'

'You do think I've got it, don't you?'

'No I don't think you've got it. Anyway, in a minute you may decide that you prefer to have the hood down.'

'What do you mean? Why would I want the hood down? I don't want a cold draught blowing around my head.'

'You'll see,' I replied, wondering how he would react when he realised he would have to sit with Ephraim's basket on his lap. The basket itself wasn't exactly spotless and certainly not germ-free, and I was expecting a volatile reaction from Richard at the prospect of nursing a dozen pigeons all the way to Dorchester.

'What's that?' he demanded.

'It's a basket of racing pigeons. We're going to release them in Dorchester.'

'Can't you put them somewhere else? How am I supposed to get in the car with that on the seat?'

'I'm afraid there isn't anywhere else to put them; the basket is too big to go in the boot. If you get in the car I'll hand the basket to you and you can sit with it.'

'I'm sorry, Justin, but I can't possibly risk touching that basket – it doesn't look clean and I shall be breathing in dust and exhaled air from the pigeons because I shall be so close to them. It isn't hygienic. No, I can't possibly do that.'

'It won't hurt you. You can wash your hands when you get to the hospital.'

'But I shall be breathing in their germs. You can catch something awful from pigeons, can't you? What is it? Psittacosis? Yes, that's it. Psittacosis – that's a terrible disease.'

'You get psittacosis from parrots not pigeons.'

51

'Do you? Well I'm sure you can catch something equally horrible from pigeons.'

'I've never heard of anybody catching anything from pigeons. Anyway, I've promised Ephraim, my landlord, that I'll take them to Dorchester and release them there. Do you want to come with me or not?'

'If I tie a handkerchief around my nose and mouth it will act like a face mask but there's still the problem of the draught with the hood down. On the other hand, if you put the hood up there'll be a greater concentration of germs in the air around me.'

'So what's worse, catching a cold or contracting some horrible fatal illness through breathing in air contaminated by pigeons?' I retorted with exasperation.

'Oh I don't know. Perhaps I'll drive myself to Dorchester and let you take the pigeons on your own.'

'Come on, Richard, don't be ridiculous. You won't catch anything from twelve perfectly fit and healthy young racing pigeons. Get in the car and let's get going.'

'Just wait a minute, I'll go and get a hat and a scarf to tie round my face. If I wear a handkerchief over my nose and mouth underneath the scarf I should be well protected.'

'So the hood stays down?'

'Yes, that will give better air circulation. Wait there I won't be long.'

He went back into his house for a good ten minutes. Finally he emerged and having checked five or six times that the door was properly locked he announced that he was ready to depart.

Looking at Richard's head, you would have thought he was about to scale Everest. He wore a thick knitted woolly hat pulled down over his forehead and he had a navy blue scarf tied around his face. Only his eyes were visible. He was carrying a travel rug, which was to serve two purposes: to prevent his legs from getting cold and to protect him from any noxious substances that might be excreted from the basket. He was also wearing a pair of bright yellow rubber gloves.

'Are you sure you'll be able to breathe under all that?' I enquired, thinking that his appearance and behaviour were absolutely ludicrous. 'At least your concerns about tetanus and catching a cold will fade into insignificance if you suffocate yourself.'

His reply was so muffled I wasn't sure what he said but I think he was indicating that he could breathe perfectly well. I lifted the basket out of the car and Richard lowered himself into the passenger seat, meticulously arranging the rug in several layers over his knees. The scarf prevented me from witnessing his expression as I placed the basket of pigeons on his lap but I had a good idea he was still not entirely happy about the situation in spite of all the protective clothing. Finally we set off for Dorchester hospital.

CHAPTER NINE

I stopped the car in a lay-by just before we reached Dorchester. Richard had hardly said a word throughout the journey and just sat rigidly in his seat holding his head high and as far away from the pigeons as possible. Although I couldn't see his face I could tell he was thankful to be rid of his feathered cargo as I lifted the basket from his lap and set it on the ground. I opened the lid and within seconds all the birds were in flight, hopefully on their way back to Luccombury. Now that the basket was empty, I was able to wedge it on its side behind the seats, much to Richard's relief, though he did not remove his scarf, hat or gloves until we got to the hospital.

The casualty department was fairly quiet with only a handful of people in the waiting room. I walked up to the receptionist who was a middle aged, somewhat overweight lady with enormous glasses.

'Good evening, I was wondering if I could get a tetanus injection, I was bitten by a dog over the weekend and I don't think I've ever had a tetanus injection before.'

'Do you need treatment for the dog bite?' she asked.

'I don't think so; it was only a small bite and I've kept it covered. I think it's all right.'

Without much enthusiasm, she began to ask me some personal details, which she wrote down on the appropriate form and when I told her I was a dentist, in reply to her enquiry as to my occupation, her manner changed immediately and she became much friendlier.

'You're a dentist, are you? I have to go and see mine at the end of the week. I'm dreading it.'

'It's never as bad as you think; I'm sure you'll be fine.'

'I've got to have a root treatment. I've never had one before and I've heard it's excruciatingly painful.'

'No it isn't. He'll give you an injection and you won't feel a thing.'

'I hope you're right.'

'There's absolutely no reason at all why dentistry should be painful. It used to be, years ago, and for some reason the memories still linger, but not any more.'

'You're very reassuring.'

'Don't worry about it. As I said, you won't feel a thing.'

She smiled at me as if I had taken a load off her mind. 'Please take a seat in the waiting area, Mr Derwent. We'll try not to keep you waiting too long.'

I moved away from the desk and Richard approached her. 'I need a tetanus injection as well,' he announced.

'Are you a dentist?' she enquired.

'No I'm a solicitor.'

She made no comment about Richard's profession but judging by the way she slipped back into her previous grouchiness, it appeared his legal credentials did not impress her. 'So were you also bitten by this dog?'

'No, I wasn't bitten by a dog.'

'So what's the problem?'

'I hurt myself gardening.'

'What was the nature of the injury?'

'I think I might have stuck a rose thorn in my finger.'

'Think? Aren't you sure? Did it bleed much?'

'No, it didn't really bleed but it was quite painful.'

'When did it happen?'

'Saturday.'

'Show me your finger.'

Richard held out his hand and the receptionist examined it closely. 'I can't see anything. From what you have told me, and from what I can see, the skin doesn't appear to have been punctured. I don't think you need a tetanus injection for that. If you want a prophylactic injection to boost your immunity, then I suggest you contact your doctor.'

'But it could be serious. It was very painful at the time and I felt very hot on Sunday,' Richard protested. 'I really think I need an injection.'

'Well, I don't think you do,' the receptionist insisted. 'Now if you'll excuse me, I have to get on with my work.'

Richard quickly accepted that it was pointless arguing with her so he came and sat down next to me, looking utterly deflated and extremely worried, but it seemed he wasn't prepared to let the matter rest.

'I'm not at all sure she's qualified to decide whether or not I need an injection; she's not a doctor. I've a good mind to go and tell her I shall be instituting legal proceedings against her, and the hospital, for breach of duty of care.'

'In order to succeed in a legal action, don't you have to prove that you've suffered as a result of the breach?' I submitted, relying on my limited knowledge of medical negligence.

'Yes, you do, but I don't suppose she'll know that and there is a real danger that I will suffer.'

'You'll have a strong case against them if you get tetanus.'

'Fat lot of good that will be when I'm dead,' Richard replied sulkily. 'How is it they are perfectly happy to give you an injection, but I've got to go and see my doctor?'

'My being a dentist might have something to do with it. We workers in the National Health Service tend to stick together and help each other out.'

'Well I'm not at all happy about the way I've been treated here. I think it's diabolical.'

No sooner had he uttered the words than his spirits were suddenly lifted by the sight of a pretty young nurse, who appeared from one of the side rooms.

'Cor, look at that,' he exclaimed, 'she's absolutely gorgeous. I'll bet she could teach me a thing or two about the workings of the human body and I wouldn't say no to her giving me a bed bath.' He continued to gaze at her as she moved around the room. 'That is definitely worth taking to the Court of Appeal – no doubt about it! Hey, did you see that? She looked over here and I'm sure there was a flicker of a smile on her face. I think she might be interested.'

'Come off it, Richard, I didn't see her smile and even if she did she was probably just being pleasant. You seem to think that every woman who as much as glances in your direction, must fancy you.'

'There, she looked this way again. I'm sure she's interested. I'm very rarely wrong about these things.'

'I think you're talking rubbish. She's probably a very pleasant girl who smiles at all the patients to make them feel better about being in the casualty department. Most people are here because they have a problem of some sort and to be greeted by a friendly smiling face helps to cheer them up. She's simply doing her job and for you to think she must fancy you just because she glanced in this direction is frankly ridiculous. She was probably looking in our direction because she knew we'd just arrived and was making a mental note of who is waiting to be treated.'

'You can think what you like, Justin, but I know enough about women and the way they behave to be able to say that she's interested, without any shadow of a doubt.'

'Do you intend to do anything about it?'

'I'm thinking about it. I certainly wouldn't mind, because she's cracking. Don't you agree?'

'She's very attractive.'

'Mr Derwent,' came the announcement from another more elderly nurse who poked her head out of a side room. 'Would you like to come this way?'

I responded to the call and left Richard still drooling over the young nurse who was speaking to one of the other patients in the waiting area. I was led into the side room and felt slightly honoured that it was not simply one of the curtained cubicles, though I don't suppose there was any particular significance in this.

'Take a seat, Mr Derwent.'

I sat down and the nurse began preparing my injection but before she was able to administer it, another nurse came into the room. 'Can you come and help for a moment, Jean, we have a slight problem in cubicle four.'

'Sorry about this, Mr Derwent, I'll be back very soon.'

I was left looking at the plain, cream walls of the treatment room. The characteristic smell of a hospital pervaded my nostrils; it was fresh, penetrating and pungently antiseptic. It was very different from the smell of a dental surgery and to my mind, far more intimidating, but to the average person both smells were probably equally objectionable. There was a high level of clinical clutter but this did not detract from the assurance of surgical sterility.

It was some ten minutes before the nurse reappeared, apologising for keeping me waiting. She promptly, and painlessly, completed the injection and announced that I was free to go. I returned to where Richard was sitting, expecting him to stand up and follow me out of the hospital.

'Hold on, Justin, I'm getting my tetanus injection after all.' He declared somewhat haughtily. 'They said they'd be ready for me very soon, if I cared to wait.'

'How the hell did you manage that?'

'I chatted up the little nurse – Denise is her name. I offered to take her out to dinner tomorrow evening if she could arrange for me to get an injection.'

'And she did?'

'Absolutely. I told you she was interested so I called her over and turned on the Darcy charm and she responded like a dream.'

'I don't believe it.' I gasped, 'If you'd told me you were intending to do that I would have said you hadn't a cat in hell's chance of succeeding.'

'It just goes to show. Never underestimate the power of the Darcy charm.'

Moments later the same nurse who had given me my injection called Richard into her room and he strutted off to join her, looking like the cat that got the cream.

I was absolutely amazed that he had managed to win over the young nurse in such a short time. I had to hand it to him that when it came to chatting up women he was a master. I couldn't help wondering, however, if the nurse would have considered him to be quite so dashing and debonair if she'd seen him sitting in my car with his woolly hat, scarf and rubber gloves, frightened to death that he might catch some awful disease from a few racing pigeons.

The other thing that puzzled me slightly was that he never seemed to strike up a long-term relationship with any of the women he met. My limited experience of women had led me to the conclusion that generally speaking, women were usually looking for lasting relationships and that once a friendship was established it wasn't easy to break it in the way that Richard did – at least, not without causing considerable upset. Perhaps he did upset the women in his life and didn't care about it, though once or twice, we had bumped into one of his previous conquests and they never seemed to bear any malice towards him, which tended to suggest that he had not treated them too badly. Perhaps the reason why the relationships had not lasted was because the women soon saw another side to him – a side which resulted in disillusionment and disappointment causing them to pull out. Richard always gave me the impression that all he was looking for was a good time, strictly on a short-term basis. I wasn't entirely convinced that this was the truth. Someone who pursued women with his vigour and enthusiasm surely had to have something more in mind than an endless series of casual encounters.

My thoughts were interrupted by the sight of Richard emerging from the treatment room. He was laughing and joking with the nurse who had administered his injection and I felt quite sure he was flirting with her, in spite of the fact that she was nearly old enough to be his mother. He crossed the waiting area to speak briefly with Denise and gave her a broad smile, which she returned. He and I then left the hospital.

CHAPTER TEN

I was very relieved to hear from Ephraim next day that all the pigeons had got back safely.

'Most o' them got back afore 'ee,' he stated with some pride. 'I saw 'ee arrive back – not sure what time 'twud be, but all but three were already 'avin' zummat t'eat in shed. Last three came in soon after. I der reckon it were pretty good fer a first flight. I'm hopin' fer great things from one or two of 'em. Let me know if 'ee intends travellin' anywhere soon an' 'ee can take a basket wi' ' ee. 'Tis good they der get practice like.'

'Sure Ephraim, I'd be happy to take them with me. I'll let you know if I'm going anywhere.'

He waved in acknowledgement and disappeared into his pigeon loft whilst Nellie sat down outside to wait patiently for him to re-emerge. I had never seen her attempt to go for the birds whilst they were outside the loft, even when they were on the ground quite close to her, but whether she could be trusted not to chase them inside the loft I wasn't sure. Ephraim obviously wasn't going to risk any of his prize birds being attacked, so Nellie had to remain outside.

The week passed amazingly quickly and as five o'clock on Friday afternoon approached I began to feel very sad because I knew that Ingrid's time at the practice had come to an end. The last patient left and whilst she was finishing clearing away I was preparing to say goodbye to her and wish her well.

'You'll be surprised to hear, Justin that you haven't quite got rid of me yet because I've agreed to come in tomorrow and help you and Spencer decorate the new waiting room.'

I was astounded. 'Did Spencer ask you to come in?'

'Yes he did. He didn't pressurize me; he just asked if there was any possibility I might still be around tomorrow and that he'd very much appreciate it if I would be willing to help out. I love decorating so I agreed to come in and do some painting.'

'He's got a cheek but I'm really pleased I'll be able to spend another day with you before you leave. Is Beryl coming in as well?'

'No I don't think so; she's going somewhere.'

'See you tomorrow then, Ingrid.'

When next morning arrived I had a strong feeling of guilt because I had not contacted Sarah. I'd promised to phone her during the week and I hadn't done so. I'd thought about her a lot but somehow I just hadn't got around to picking up the phone, so did that say something about my feelings towards her? Surely if I'd been keen I would have made the effort to get in touch. I think the truth was that I wanted to see her but I was slightly apprehensive about appearing too keen and giving her the wrong impression. Perhaps I needed some lessons from Richard Darcy on how to handle women.

I had arranged to go to the practice at around ten o'clock, so I decided to phone Sarah before I set out.

'Hello, Justin, how lovely to hear from you. Are you all right?'

'Yes, fine thank you, Sarah, how are you?'

'Very well, thank you. I've been thinking about you all week, hoping you'd phone.'

'I'm sorry I didn't manage to phone earlier but you know how it is.'

'Of course, you don't have to apologise. I'm just so pleased you've phoned now. What are you doing today?'

'I'm going to the practice to help with some decorating. We're going to move the surgeries downstairs. It's quite exciting because it means we'll be installing new equipment. Heaven knows it's about time – the gear we have at present is ancient.'

'That's exciting. Have you designed your new surgery yet?'

'No, not yet. Spencer has only just made the decision to reorganise the practice. It's still early days and I haven't really had time to think about it. Anyway, what are you doing today?'

'Not a lot, really. I may go shopping later on but I haven't really any definite plans.'

'I was wondering if you would like to go for a drive tomorrow morning and perhaps we could go for a pub lunch somewhere.'

'That would be really nice, Justin; I'd love to.'

'Great, so will it be all right if I pick you up about ten?'

'Whatever time you say, I'll be ready. Oh, by the way, how is your hand where Tigger bit you? I wanted to phone and ask you about it but I didn't like to, in case you thought I was badgering you. You said you'd phone me so I thought I'd better wait until you did, but I've been very concerned about you.'

'It's fine. It was only a little scratch – nothing at all to worry about.'

'That's good. I was most upset about it. I'll let you get on with your decorating now and look forward to seeing you tomorrow. Actually there is something I want to talk to you about, but I'll let it wait until tomorrow.'

'Ten o'clock then, Sarah, bye.'

'Goodbye, Justin, and thank you.'

I put down the phone, pleased that I had invited Sarah out. Hearing her voice made me realise that I did want to be with her and taking her out for lunch and going for a walk in the country or by the sea would be a very pleasant way to spend my Sunday. I wondered what it could be she wanted to talk to me about – I really had no idea and I was more than a little bit intrigued but no doubt I would soon find out.

With these thoughts in mind, I drove round to Fothergill House where Ingrid and Spencer were already hard at work in what would be the new waiting room. Spencer had obviously been working on it in the evenings and I was amazed at what he'd already achieved. The walls were no longer oily. Apparently there had been some sort of paper on them and by stripping this off, which Spencer had done completely; most of the oil had been eliminated. He had plastered the holes and filled all the defects so the room was now ready for painting. He had addressed the problem of the oily floorboards with a combination of scrubbing and sanding, and whilst they weren't exactly pristine, they were greatly improved.

'I would have liked to have left the floorboards uncovered and just polish them,' he proclaimed. 'I was hoping I could avoid the expense of carpet but unfortunately I don't think I'll be able to get away with it; there are places where I just couldn't shift the oil and it wouldn't look very good.'

'Carpet will be much warmer,' Ingrid commented. 'There are some quite wide gaps between the boards and you can feel the draught coming up from underneath.'

'That's true,' Spencer admitted. 'It's slightly unusual for a house of this age to have a suspended floor; usually the floors are solid, often with flagstones. I'm not sure if it was always like this or whether the solid floors were dug out and timber put in later. In Daphne's office there's a trap door, which enables you go under the floor. You can crawl around down there and get to any part of the house. The space under the floors is about four feet deep and will be very useful when we move the surgeries downstairs – we can run the plumbing and the wiring in the space.'

The three of us set about transforming the room. Ingrid and I began painting the walls with a nondescript shade of cream emulsion paint or maybe it was actually distemper. It obviously wasn't new paint because the tin was rusting quite badly around the lid and it was impossible to read the label because it was so old and dirty.

'Where did you get the paint from, Spencer?' I asked.

'I'm not sure where it came from originally. It's been lying around in my outside workshop for as long as I can remember. I nearly threw it out on several occasions but I kept thinking it might come in useful one day and it would be a shame to waste perfectly good paint. It's all right, isn't it?'

'It's a bit watery. The walls will need a good few coats to cover properly.'

'That's all right,' he said, 'there's plenty of it. There are at least another two tins out there if you need them. I think they're all the same colour.'

'Don't you think it would be a good idea to check now? If they aren't all the same, it's going to look a bit odd if the walls are all different.'

'I'm pretty sure all the tins contain the same colour paint. In any case, people aren't likely to notice if there's a slight difference. In my experience, they are generally very unobservant.'

Spencer finished preparing the woodwork for painting and produced a tin of some sort of oil-based paint. It was also cream, though it didn't appear to be quite the same shade as the emulsion Ingrid and I were using, but it was every bit as ancient.

'The patients will probably get lead poisoning from the paint you're using, Spencer,' I joked.

'Nonsense,' he replied. 'This is decent paint – not like the rubbish you buy today. It may well have lead in it but that's what makes it so good. The patients aren't exactly going to be eating it, are

63

they? It's perfectly safe and the great thing is that this woodwork will probably never need painting again – not in our lifetime anyway. You wouldn't be able to say that if you were using modern paint.'

'So where did you buy it from?' Ingrid enquired with a grin, knowing full well he wouldn't have bought it.

'My father had it in his garage; he bought it for something and never used it so I thought I might as well make use of it.'

'Lucky it's nearly the same colour as the walls,' I chuckled. 'What colour carpet are you intending to fit?'

'I'm not quite sure yet,' said Spencer.

'Depends what he can get hold of without having to pay for it,' Ingrid whispered to me, though I suspect Spencer caught the gist of what she was saying.

'I believe in making use of things which would otherwise be thrown away, especially when they are of good quality. I can't bear waste and there aren't many new things that impress me. Nothing seems to be made to last anymore. I'm looking for good solid workmanship which, sadly, only appears to be found in things that were made years ago.'

'Like with dental equipment?' I asked, wondering if Spencer had yet found any equipment that had excited him sufficiently for him to want to install it in his new surgery.

'Exactly,' he retorted. 'I have to say I haven't seen any modern equipment that looks really well made and will have long-term reliability. To my mind it's like modern cars – very flashy and attractive on the surface but not built to last.

'Have you looked at German-made equipment? I've heard that it's generally well-made and more reliable than most,' I remarked.

Ingrid was quick to back me up. 'Most things made in Germany are good, Spencer. Much better than you make here in Britain.'

'Mm,' he replied without conviction.

'Well, you'll need to make your mind up soon, Spencer; we're making rapid progress here. This waiting room will soon be up and running and you'll need to have your new equipment sorted out. Without it you won't be able to set up your surgery downstairs. I know you want to move as soon as possible.'

'Yes I do, you're right.'

By five o'clock, we had virtually finished the decorating. There were just one or two finishing touches needed, which Spencer said he would complete next day. I thought the room actually looked quite smart, though perhaps I was comparing it with how it looked a week previously, rather than judging it objectively. Surprisingly, the slight mismatch in colour between the walls and the woodwork didn't seem to matter and in spite off the fact that Ingrid and I had had to use three tins of emulsion paint, the walls all appeared to look more or less the same.

'As soon as I get some carpet, we'll be away,' Spencer declared. 'I'm really pleased with the way this room looks and thank you both for your help. What we've achieved today marks the beginning of a new era for our practice I'm just sorry that Ingrid won't be a part of it any longer. We're moving forward and bringing about improvements, which will greatly benefit our patients, provide us with greater job satisfaction, and also make the practice of dentistry considerably more lucrative. I realise now that we've been standing still for too long, but that is now coming to an end and very soon we'll see a different class of patient filling our appointment books. There are exciting times ahead; I'm convinced of it.'

It was a stirring speech from Spencer but I couldn't help thinking it was completely out of character. Ever since I first met him, he had made it clear he was quite happy to muddle along in a simple way and the idea of spending money on updating his practice had, until now, been completely alien to him. Had Lady Gascoyne-Fairley and the prospect of adding some of her wealthy friends to his list of patients really motivated him to such an extent that he'd had a complete rethink on his way of running the practice? At the risk of being over-cynical, I decided that I would believe it when I saw more evidence.

Spencer insisted we had a cup of tea before we left and we sat in his kitchen munching our way through some delicious biscuits that Daphne had baked. We had hardly mentioned Ingrid's leaving all day and it was almost as if we were all wishing it wasn't going to happen. However, when she announced that the time had come for her to go home it was a very emotional moment.

'We and the patients are going to miss you very much and if I thought I could persuade you to change your mind I would certainly try but I understand your reasons for leaving and I respect them,' said Spencer. He kissed and hugged her and I did the same.

'Take care of yourself, Ingrid and thank you for all your help. It's been a real pleasure to have you as my nurse.'

There were tears in her eyes as she put on her coat and opened the front door of the practice. She had one quick glance behind her and stepped out into the world to enter a new chapter in her life.

CHAPTER ELEVEN

When I looked out of my window next morning, I couldn't help noticing some large pools of water in the garden – water that had collected overnight, as a result of some very heavy and prolonged bouts of rain. The weather had turned very unsettled and it did not look at all promising for a walk in the country or by the sea. I felt sure, however, that Sarah would not mind in the least and I was looking forward to our day together, even though we might have to modify our plans somewhat.

My drive to Sarah's house took me in a northerly direction up a long and, at times, steep road. Looking back, there were spectacular views over the entire town and surrounding area, with the church and its magnificent tower dominating the landscape. The road was appropriately named 'Tunnel Road' because about a mile and a half from the town centre there was an impressive road tunnel some twenty feet high, and twenty feet wide, taking the road through a large and otherwise insurmountable hill. It was a little over a hundred yards in length and local people maintained that weather conditions were frequently completely different on each side of the tunnel. I was highly sceptical about it but as I emerged on the northern side, there was no doubt that I was looking at some blue sky ahead of me, and the clouds were much less menacing. Perhaps there was some truth in the local belief.

By the time I reached Sarah's house, the rain had stopped but judging by the clouds in the distance, and if the weather forecast was anything to go by, it seemed unlikely that the dry conditions would last very long. Sarah was ready and waiting for me at her front door and I got out of my car to greet her.

'It's lovely to see you, Justin,' Sarah said, throwing her arms around me.

'I don't know if we'll be able to go for a walk today unless we're prepared to get soaked,' I remarked.

'I don't mind at all,' Sarah replied. 'I'm happy to walk in the rain if you want to, though I don't think either of us is wearing the right clothes for it.'

'Why don't we head for the coast and hope that the weather clears sufficiently to allow us to go for a walk by the sea. If it doesn't, we could watch the sea, which might be quite rough. I've got my camera with me and there could be a chance to take some dramatic photographs.'

'Fine by me,' agreed Sarah. 'By the way, are you sure your hand is all right where Tigger bit you?'

'It's perfectly all right. She only just broke the skin and it's more or less healed up now. I did go for a tetanus injection though, just to be on the safe side.'

'Probably wise if you haven't had one recently. When did you go?'

'I went to Dorchester hospital on Monday evening. Richard Darcy, a friend of mine went with me and he had an injection as well.'

'Richard Darcy?' exclaimed Sarah in a disapproving tone.

'Yes, do you know him?'

'I've only met him once – he tried to pick me up. But I've heard a lot about him.'

'Really?'

'He's a womaniser!'

I felt I had to come to Richard's defence. 'I wouldn't say that. It's true that he's constantly looking for women. He likes taking them out and impressing them with his Oxford education and his position as a solicitor. He meets someone, takes her out a few times then moves on to someone else.'

'He treats them very badly. As you say, he impresses them, sweeps them off their feet and then drops them again just as quickly. He never seems to stay with the same girl for more than a few weeks. I really don't know what he's looking for but surely he should know by now that he's looking in the wrong places if he wants to find a long-term partner. I personally think he's on some sort of ego trip and doesn't want a proper relationship. He just gets a kick out of chatting up gullible women and making them think he's wonderful.'

'I'm not sure what he's looking for, either. I think he just enjoys the chase but I don't think he makes any promises to the girls he meets. I would say he's pretty harmless really.'

'Well I don't, Justin. I don't like what I've heard about him and I don't want you associating with him – I think he's a bad influence.'

'He's a friend, Sarah. He's a bit odd at times and has some rather peculiar ways but none of us is perfect. He was the first person to befriend me when I came to live in Luccombury and in spite of his eccentricity I quite like him. I suppose I feel sorry for him in a way, because it may be that he's looking for a special companion – maybe even a wife and, if he is, then it must be frustrating for him that he can't seem to find the right person.'

'Well he isn't likely to find the right person in the sort of places he frequents. He's supposed to be intelligent, so he should be aware of that. The fact that he goes looking in these places suggests to me that he isn't looking for a long term partner; he just wants to meet girls he can take advantage of. I'm not at all happy about you going out with him, Justin, I'd rather you didn't.'

I wasn't prepared to promise Sarah that I wouldn't see Richard again and to some extent I resented her attempt to control my choice of friends. I found him witty and amusing. Admittedly, sometimes it was a case of laughing at him rather than with him but he was aware of this and didn't seem to mind at all. Personally I couldn't share his obsession for going out to pick up women but that was the way he was and I accepted it even though I didn't necessarily agree with it. To me the essence of friendship is taking people as they are, even if their ways aren't the same as one's own. I decided it would be wise not to say any more about him to Sarah and I put my mind to searching for a new topic of discussion to divert her attention.

To get to the coast we had to travel back the way I had come, returning through the tunnel and this gave me a good opportunity to change the subject. 'Did you know that the local people claim that the weather is often completely different on each side of this tunnel?'

'I've heard that,' replied Sarah, 'it has to be rubbish, doesn't it?'

'I would have thought so, though many locals firmly believe it.'

As we emerged on the south side it was apparent that on this occasion local superstition was wrong and the weather was exactly the same as on the north side – dry at present, but with clouds gathering all round us and getting blacker by the minute. We pressed on towards the sea and soon it became so dark I had to put my lights on.

It was like a total eclipse of the sun – black as night. The wind, which had been whipping up fallen leaves, suddenly dropped creating an eerie stillness and a very strong sensation of impending doom. If someone had told me the world was about to end, I would have believed it.

'This is amazing,' said Sarah who seemed quite excited about the extreme weather conditions we were experiencing.'

'It's weird, isn't it? I don't think I've ever seen it go so dark during the day. I'm sure I can see the Four Horsemen of the Apocalypse in that field over there.'

'I imagine the end of the world could be like this,' Sarah opined, 'but I feel sure that this is nothing more than a spot of bad weather.'

'I hope you're right, I'm not ready to meet my maker just yet.'

We watched in awe, as the entire world seemed to stand still in anticipation of something happening. It might just be a spot of bad weather but I certainly hadn't seen anything quite so disturbing before. The stillness was so intense, it was almost unbearable and lingered for some minutes, then the calmness was shattered dramatically, as the entire sky was illuminated for a split second by an intensely bright streak of lightning, which carved a jagged path before our very eyes, and the spine-chilling silence was blown apart by a terrific peal of thunder. A few moments later, the heavens opened and hailstones as big as golf balls hurtled down upon us. The elasticity in the hood of my car was tested to its limit by the impact of the hailstones, which bounced off it like youngsters on a trampoline.

I was afraid the hood would not be able to withstand this level of bombardment for very long but there seemed to be no means of escape. Then I remembered that just around the next bend was a bridge across the road. I made a dash for it, stopped the car underneath and waited for the storm to pass. Mine was not the only car under the bridge – there was a small red saloon also taking shelter from the hailstones and the distraught owner was inspecting his roof. I got out of my car to check for damage, fortunately there didn't appear to be any but the red saloon had not been so lucky as there were several quite noticeable dents in the metal of the roof and the bonnet.

'I've never seen anything like it,' grumbled the agitated driver, struggling in the dim light to assess the extent of the damage to his otherwise very shiny and unmarked red car.

'It's unbelievable weather, I know the weather forecast was not good but I don't think they predicted anything quite as bad as this.'

'Blooming weather forecast – it's useless, I don't know why I bother listening.' The unfortunate motorist was well and truly disgruntled and I could understand how he felt. Repairing his car would not be easy and would no doubt prove expensive.

It was about ten minutes before the storm eased and we set off once again on our journey. The road was covered with the balls of ice, which were beginning to melt creating an extremely slippery surface. Driving was downright hazardous so we decided to head for a garden centre situated near Westport and stop there for a cup of coffee.

'A cup of coffee would go down very well,' said Sarah, who seemed completely unruffled by the circumstances. The fact that we had nearly skidded off the road didn't appear to have worried her one little bit.

'We can wait there until the roads are clear of ice.' I suggested. 'It shouldn't take long – it's melting quite quickly.'

The sky still looked menacing and I was worried about leaving my car out in the open in case there was another hailstorm. By pure chance, there were some vacant parking spaces under a wooden pergola, which would at least offer some protection, though it was not complete cover. We went into the garden centre and made for the coffee shop. It seemed that many people had the same idea because the place was quite full but we managed to find a vacant table in a corner and sat down to enjoy what I thought would be a very welcome drink after the ordeal we had just experienced.

I had barely taken two sips when there was another terrific crash of thunder followed by a further deluge from the sky. It wasn't hailstones this time but torrential rain on a scale that was simply unimaginable. My first thought was to be thankful we were under cover but what I didn't know was that the roof of the coffee shop, which was constructed of some sort of plastic material, had been damaged by the previous hailstones, allowing water to collect above the ceiling. As I looked up, I could see great bulges appearing and before I, or anyone else could take evasive action, the ceiling split open in three or four places pouring gallons of water onto the unfortunate individuals sitting underneath.

Sarah and I, being in a corner, managed to avoid the worst of the cascade, though we didn't escape entirely unscathed. Compared with those sitting in the middle of the room, however, we got off very lightly. Utter pandemonium ensued as everyone made a dive for the exit but the problem was that the rain was still bucketing down so there was little point in going outside. The only other way out was into the adjoining sales area but the roof in there had suffered a similar fate so that was flooded too, with water gushing down from gaping holes in the ceiling. People were screaming and shouting and rushing around in complete panic.

'Best stay where we are at the moment,' said Sarah who still appeared completely unruffled. She picked up her cup of coffee and went to stand close to the wall where it was relatively dry. 'We'll wait here and let the hysteria die down.'

'What a day this is turning out to be, I hope my car's all right,' I said anxiously.

'It'll be fine, Justin, you worry too much. It might be a bit wet inside but it'll dry out. It's exciting when things like this happen, don't you think? Life would be very dull if everything was perfect all the time.'

'I suppose you're right,' I uttered doubtfully.

Eventually the rain eased off, the room gradually cleared of customers and the members of staff set about sweeping out the water and clearing up the considerable mess. It would take some time before the garden centre was functioning normally again and the threat of further similar downpours remained. Sarah finished her coffee and we went out to find my car. I was very apprehensive about the state I would find it in but as it turned out, the hood had done a magnificent job of keeping the interior dry. Apart from a few splashes on the inside of the doors there was no evidence that that any water had penetrated.

'Phew, what a relief,' I sighed.

'I told you it would be all right. Let's go into Westport now. The wind is getting up again and the sea should be quite rough. I love it when it's really wild and the spray is blowing everywhere.'

CHAPTER TWELVE

We set off on our way once again to find, not surprisingly, that there was a tremendous amount of water on the road and in places there were deep puddles. We pressed on at a very modest pace because all the cars heading for Westport, having previously been held up by the weather, were now on the move so traffic was very heavy, particularly for a Sunday morning.

'If you take the next left,' Sarah exclaimed, 'we'll avoid this traffic. You go along for a couple of miles and then take a sharp right and double back into Westport. It's a bit further but progress is so slow on the main road it will be just as quick in the long run.'

'I don't know that road.'

'I often take it. It's usually very quiet, though a bit narrow in places.'

I did as Sarah suggested and was thankful to be off the main road and out of the line of cars, which seemed to be playing follow-my-leader at a snail's pace.

'A little drop of rain and the world virtually grinds to a standstill,' she scoffed. 'Why are they all driving so slowly?'

Sarah's description that the road was a bit narrow in places was not entirely accurate. It was, in fact, little more than the width of my tiny car for most of the way, though there were some passing places. There were also many very sharp bends. We travelled on for about a mile when I saw that there was a considerable amount of water on the road ahead of me. I slowed down trying to assess the likely depth of the flood before risking taking my little sports car through it.

'I don't think you need worry, Justin. As I said, I often come this way and from what I can remember of this stretch of road I'm pretty sure the water is no more than a few inches deep. I'm going by that fence over there – I can see the bottom of the posts.' Sarah sounded confident and reassuring so I took her word for it and pressed forward gingerly. The flood extended for a good thirty feet along the road and for the first fifteen or so we were fine – the water was no more than a couple of inches deep. Unfortunately, there must have been a submerged dip in the road and suddenly we found ourselves in deeper water. The engine misfired and spluttered several times before dying completely.

'I'm sorry, Justin,' Sarah whispered, looking very guilty that she had been responsible for suggesting that it would be safe to press on into the flood.

'You weren't to know there would be a dip in the road. The water isn't all that deep, but my car is very low. The question is – what the hell do we do now?' I wasn't exactly pleased with her for urging me on into the water and she was the one who suggested we came this way, but after all, it was I who made the final decision to try to drive through the water.

'I'll have to push us out. You stay here. There's no point in both of us getting our feet wet. I think I'll push it back rather than forward, the water might get even deeper further on.'

'You can't push it on your own. I'll get out and help you.' And with that she opened her door, which allowed water to gush into the car interior.

I sighed in exasperation. 'I was going to put down the hood and climb out over the door because I knew what would happen if I opened the door.'

'Oh Justin, I'm so sorry, I didn't think the water was above the bottom of the door. I'm not doing very well, am I? You won't want to go out with me again after this.'

I didn't answer and although there was now a considerable amount of water in the car, I decided that opening my door would only add to it so I pushed back the hood and climbed out. The water was freezing cold and immediately filled my shoes. I paddled to the front of the car and tried to push it but the road surface was very slippery and my efforts were in vain. Sarah was pushing as well but even our combined force seemed to be making no impact on the stranded vehicle. The problem was that we were unable to gain sufficient momentum to get it out of the distinct dip in the road. We pushed and strained for some minutes until we were both exhausted. Then we heard a voice calling to us.

'I reckon if they'd intended yer to take it to water, they'd 'ave fitted it with a rudder and propeller.' I looked up to see a big round face smiling back at me from the field at the side of the road. 'You bain't be the first to come to grief just there – that bit o' road often floods. If you 'ang on a minute I'll go and get my tractor and tow 'im out.'

'Thank you so much,' I shouted back. 'I don't think we'll be able to push it out ourselves.'

'Don't worry, I'll soon 'ave 'im out. Wait there, I'll be back in a minute.'

It wasn't long before a huge tractor appeared out of a gate further down the road. It was so big it looked as though it could easily go through six feet of water without any difficulty. The jovial farmer jumped out and waded into the water to attach a tow rope to the back of my car and in no time at all, my prize possession was returned to relatively dry land.

'What do yer wanna do wi'n now?' he asked, 'I don't think yer'll be driving 'im anywhere today.'

'I really don't know,' I replied dejectedly, 'I suppose I shall have to get a garage to come out and fetch it so that they can get it going again.'

'Well yer can't really leave 'im 'ere, yer blockin' th'road. Cars that aren't as low-slung as yours could as like get through the flood but they won't be able to if yer leave your car there. I suggests you let me tow 'im back to my house and I'll get missus ter make you a cup o' tea. Then we'll 'ave a go at drying 'im out and see if we can get 'im started.'

'That's extremely kind of you.'

'I be Arthur. Nice to meet yer,' he said amiably, holding out a wet hand.

'I'm Justin and this is Sarah, thank you so much for helping us.'

'You follow me back. House is only just down th' road.'

Sarah and I were conscious of the fact that our shoes were dripping muddy water and we took them off before going into the farmer's house.

'I'll put 'em in front of the fire to dry off a bit whilst yer drink yer tea. Go in and sit down. You'd better take yer socks off as well, I'll get yer some towels to dry yer feet.'

'I can't tell you how grateful we are. I really don't know what we'd have done without your help,' I said. 'We shouldn't have tried to drive through the flood – it was a bit stupid. I ought to have known that my car was too low.'

'It was my fault,' Sarah interjected. 'I didn't think the water was very deep and I told him to keep going. I didn't know there was a dip in the road.'

'I dare say he'll forgive yer, my dear. 'ave yer bin wed long?'

'We aren't married.'

'Noah? Well in that case 'ee's probably forgiven yer already.'

Sarah and I were grateful for the tea and we sat talking for a good three quarters of an hour before Arthur finally stood up. 'I'll go and see if I can get 'im goin'. Yer shoes and socks won't be completely dry but they won't be as wet as when yer came in. Judging by the amount of water inside yon car, yer feet be goin' to get another soaking afore yer get 'ome.'

Arthur went outside whilst Sarah and I retrieved our footwear from the fireside.

'I'm so sorry, Justin, I know how much you love your car. Please don't be angry with me.'

'It's all right, Sarah, I don't blame you. It happened and that's all there is to it. It wasn't your fault.'

We took our shoes to the door before putting them on as they were still quite wet and we didn't want to make a mess on the kitchen floor, though it was a typical farmhouse floor and looked as if it was used to getting messy. Before we had time to thank Arthur's wife for the tea, he returned with his face beaming.

'I got 'im goin'.'

I couldn't believe it. 'Really, that's fantastic. How did you manage it?'

'I jus' dried off the plug leads an' distributor cap and 'ee started up straightaway. No real 'arm done but I should avoid deep puddles if I were you.'

'Oh I will thank you, Arthur. Thank you very much and thank your wife for the tea.' I shook his hand warmly and Arthur kissed Sarah as if he'd known her for years.

Although the car was running again, the interior was extremely wet with a couple of inches of water lying over the entire floor area. The weather hadn't improved much at all with more storm clouds gathering by the minute.

'I think we are going to have to call it a day,' I declared. 'There isn't much hope of a walk and we need to change our socks and shoes.'

'We could go back to my house if you like,' Sarah suggested. 'I'll get us some lunch and we can dry off there.'

I didn't have any better ideas, so I agreed. Secretly, however, what I really wanted was to get the water out of my car and dry off the carpets but that would have to wait for the moment.

Sarah's dogs were very pleased to see us and we brightened up what for them would have been an uninteresting afternoon with only Sarah's mother to entertain them. They leapt for joy when they saw us, barking furiously and much to my amazement, Tigger kept licking my thumb – the same one she had bitten a week ago. I thought there probably wasn't any particular significance to it, but Sarah was convinced it was Tigger's way of saying she was sorry for what she'd done.

Sarah prepared us a very enjoyable lunch with cold chicken and salad and we sat with bare feet in front of the fire drinking cups of tea and reading the Sunday newspapers. It wasn't quite what we'd planned but nevertheless it was a pleasant way to spend a very gloomy afternoon. For much of the time, we sat side-by-side, occasionally holding hands but this was as far as our display of affection went. In any case, as Sarah's mother was in and out of the room all afternoon it would have been difficult to let our feelings run away, even if we'd wanted to. There was the added problem that whenever Tigger felt I was getting too close to Sarah she let out a low-pitched warning growl.

Although the temptation to languish in total relaxation was great, by five o'clock, my desire to sort out my car became overwhelming.

'I really think I ought to be going now, Sarah,' I said. 'Thank you for a wonderful lunch but there are a few things I'd like to do before tomorrow.'

'Of course,' Sarah replied, 'I understand, but please don't feel you have to go. You're more than welcome to stay as long as you like. You can stay and eat with mother and me this evening if you want to.'

'That's very sweet of you, but I really must go.'

'Before you leave, there is something I want to talk to you about.' Sarah hesitated and I became intrigued to know what it was she wanted to say to me.

'I've heard about a weekend course I'd love to go on and I wondered if you'd be prepared to come with me.'

'What sort of course?'

'Well, they train you to parachute jump. The training starts early on Saturday morning for the whole day and continues on Sunday morning and then on Sunday afternoon you go up in a plane and do your first jump. I'd love to do it, Justin, will you come with me? Please say you will. I think it will be so exciting.'

I gulped. I don't think I had ever given serious consideration to taking up parachute jumping and, to be perfectly honest; jumping out of an aircraft was not high on the list of activities I wanted to engage in.

'Wow, Sarah, whatever made you want to do that?'

'It's something I've always wanted. It must be so electrifying to feel the wind rushing past you as you look down on the world from several thousand feet and you allow gravity to pull you towards the ground, getting faster and faster, thinking that you could be heading for certain death as the land rushes upwards to meet you. But you know really that it won't happen, because your parachute will save you. You pull the cord and immediately, your speed of descent is checked as your parachute opens and you float down the rest of the way in safety. You've experienced the thrill of falling freely, out of control, and now you can enjoy gently gliding to the ground. I can't think of anything more exhilarating. Please say you'll come with me, Justin, I don't want to go on my own.'

I really didn't know what to say. I wanted to tell Sarah that the idea was ridiculous and that I had not the slightest inclination to jump out of an aircraft with or without a parachute, but she seemed so excited about it I didn't feel I could crush her enthusiasm with an out-and-out refusal right from the start.

'I can't say I've ever thought about parachute jumping, I shall need to think about it, though I have to say that I'm very apprehensive.'

'Of course you are, Justin, but that's what makes it exciting. So you aren't saying you won't do it?'

'I'm not saying I will or I won't.'

'But promise me you'll give it serious consideration. It would be so romantic to jump out of the plane together, holding hands.'

I didn't like to say that I didn't think it would be the slightest bit romantic and I wondered whether it was fair to let Sarah go on thinking that I might agree to join her in this hare-brained idea. Perhaps I should have told her, there and then, that there was no way I would ever consider jumping out of an aircraft. However I couldn't bring myself to say it at that moment. I put on my shoes and socks, kissed her and left.

'Promise me you'll think about it, Justin. It would be wonderful if you'd agree to come with me. Please say you will.'

CHAPTER THIRTEEN

The interior of my car smelt distinctly musty next morning when I set off for work. I had mopped up all the water from the floor and done my best to get as much water from the carpets as I could, but in spite of my efforts, everything was still extremely damp and would probably remain so for some time to come. At least the engine was running and didn't appear to have suffered any real damage as a result of the soaking it had received.

When I arrived at the practice, I found Spencer to be in a buoyant mood and he virtually pounced on me as soon as I set foot inside the door.

'The new waiting room is now fully operational,' he announced, with considerable self-satisfaction.

'It can't be.' I gasped in disbelief. 'There was still so much to do when I left here on Saturday. You didn't have any carpet. Surely you haven't been able to get hold of some and get it fitted in such a short time.'

'Come and see.'

Spencer wasn't renowned for his speed when it came to doing things for the practice but quite clearly, on this occasion, something was motivating him. He opened the door of the new waiting room and as I walked in, it was as if the carpet jumped off the floor and hit me.

'It's a bit busy, isn't it, Spencer?' It was predominantly green but also contained varying amounts of every colour you could think of. Huge orange and lemon swirls gyrated in a clockwise direction around the floor.

'Well, I probably wouldn't have chosen something quite so brightly coloured or with such a strong pattern if I'd been buying new, but a friend of mine offered it to me. It's been lying around in

80

his loft for some time. I needed some carpet quickly, and I thought it was too good to miss. I gave him a bottle of Scotch for it and he helped me fit it. We did it yesterday afternoon and I moved the furniture in during the evening.'

'So, we now have a new waiting room.'

'That's right, Justin. The only thing left for me to do is to transfer the sign from the door of the old waiting room to this one. I was about to do that when you arrived.'

'Well if any patients go into the old waiting room by mistake they'll soon realise that something has changed when they find the room completely bare, with no chairs to sit on.'

'A good point, Justin, but that room has always been the waiting room and I have learnt from experience that old habits die hard.'

'I can believe that. Also the new waiting room is at the back of the house whilst the old one was just inside the front door. Some patients might get lost and unless you get the signage sorted out so that they all understand where they should be going, you'll have patients wandering into your new surgery.'

'I've thought of that but they'll get used to it eventually. In any event, I'm hoping to start moving my surgery downstairs without delay. I think it's such a good idea; I can't wait to get on with it.'

'You're certainly pushing ahead with great speed, Spencer. It's not like you at all.'

'You obviously don't know me very well. When I get a really good idea, I can't rest until I've put it into operation. I'm convinced that moving downstairs will be a great improvement in lots of ways.'

'Will I be moving downstairs in the near future?'

'Yes. It's all part of the master plan, but obviously we'll have to take it one step at a time. We've completed the first step, which is to move the waiting room. The next one is to move my surgery. But don't worry, Justin, your turn will come. Just bear with me.'

I wanted to mention that I was considering the possibility of buying new equipment for my surgery but I decided there wasn't really time to discuss it at that moment. I was more concerned about my new nurse who would, or should, be arriving very shortly and I was somewhat apprehensive at the prospect.

'What time is Wendy coming?' I asked.

'I told her your first patient was at nine o'clock and she said she'd be here in good time. It's only just after eight thirty.'

'I hope she comes soon; it doesn't give her long to get to know my surgery.'

'I'm sure she'll be here. Oh, by the way, you're always saying you never get to see any young female patients because I always claim them for myself. Well, you can't say that today. Two very attractive young students came to the door just before you arrived. They are home from university and both have minor dental problems. They say they're worried and want to be seen but I don't honestly think either of them has anything seriously wrong. I've arranged to see one of them; but unfortunately, I'm too busy to see them both so I put one of them in with you this afternoon.'

'Good grief. Things are changing at this practice. But thank you, it will make a pleasant change from seeing the old fogies with their dentures.'

'Who is your first patient this morning?' Spencer asked as I edged my way towards the stairs.

'Mr Rutherford. Do you know him?'

'James Rutherford? Oh yes, I know him – he's completely balmy. He used to be an English teacher. He's constantly quoting Shakespeare or worse and never stops talking. Treating him is well-nigh impossible.'

'He hasn't been for over two years so it may be that he's got trouble, and that's why he made an appointment.'

'I wouldn't be surprised because he never, and I mean never, brushes his teeth. They are completely buried under masses of tartar. I wish you luck; you'll probably need it.'

'Thanks, Spencer.'

I started to mount the stairs when the front door burst open and a very flustered blonde girl crashed into the entrance hall. She was slim, petite, very smartly dressed and carrying three large shopping bags. In spite of her obvious agitation her eyes sparkled and she smiled sweetly when she saw Spencer. 'I'm so sorry I'm late, Mr Padginton. I know it doesn't look good on my first morning but I assure you I don't make a habit of it. I was about to leave home when I realised one of my cats was missing. One was run over by a car a few months ago and I hate leaving the house now unless I know they're safely locked in. The little rascal had managed to sneak through the back door and I had an awful job getting him in. I'm really sorry.'

'Hello, Wendy,' I called out from half way up the stairs. 'I'm very pleased to meet you.'

'You must be Mr Derwent,' she replied as we shook hands.

'We use Christian names here, Wendy. He's Justin and you must call me Spencer. You'll be nursing for him but you know that don't you? His last nurse simply couldn't stand working for him any longer and fled off back to Germany where she came from. He's almost impossible to work for. In fact, the nurse he had before her only lasted a morning. He reduced her to a complete nervous wreck in less than three hours.'

Although Spencer sounded quite serious, Wendy was completely unperturbed.

'I've worked for a few difficult dentists in my time; I expect I can handle him,' she replied and her eyes twinkled again.

'Come with me, my dear,' said Spencer, 'and I'll introduce you to Beryl and show you where you can hang your coat then Justin will take you to his surgery.'

Whilst I was waiting for Wendy to join me, the front door opened and Reverend Jenkinson entered.

'I just wanted to catch you before you started work, Justin. You'll be pleased to hear that my tooth is fine now, that "brown paste" whatever it was worked wonders. It took about twenty minutes, then the pain subsided and that was the end of it. I don't know what it is but it's marvellous stuff.'

'That's amazing,' I remarked. 'I don't know what it is either but Spencer swears by it and it certainly worked in your case when everything else I'd tried had failed.'

'I was so grateful to you for all you did for me; I felt I was becoming a bit of a nuisance having to keep coming back but I really was in a lot of pain.'

'I know you were Reverend Jenkinson and you weren't a nuisance at all. I'm just sorry I didn't know about the paste sooner.'

'Well I'm very grateful and I've brought you a little something to show my appreciation.'

He handed me a bottle of wine.

'That really is most kind of you.'

'I hope you like red wine.'

'Indeed I do and thank you very much but there was no need for you to feel you had to bring me something to show your appreciation. I'm so pleased though that we were able to stop your pain before the wedding you were conducting. That must have been a great relief for you.'

'Ah yes, the wedding.' His tone suggested it had not been the happy event one would normally expect a wedding to be. 'The less said about that the better.'

'Oh dear, was there a problem?'

'I'm afraid there was rather. It all started when I asked if anyone knew of any just cause why the couple should not be joined in matrimony and the bride's brother jumped to his feet and starting hurling abuse at the groom. He said that he wasn't good enough for her and that he was a sponging layabout who was only marrying her because he knew she had some money and was likely to inherit a good deal more when her elderly father passed away.

'That prompted an ex-girlfriend of the groom to retaliate by saying that the bride was a scheming cow who had gone out of her way to steal him from her when they were about to get engaged. She claimed that the bride had had so many men it was impossible to keep track of them all and that she couldn't be faithful to anyone for more than a few weeks and the chances of the marriage lasting were virtually non-existent. She just wished the poor sod hadn't been so besotted with her that all common sense had gone out of the window but she couldn't just sit back and watch him make an absolute fool of himself by marrying her.'

'So what happened? Did you marry them?'

'Eventually, yes. I took them into the vestry and asked if they were both sure they wanted to go ahead with the wedding. They said they were so we went back and I told the congregation that the personal feelings of individuals did not amount to "just cause why the couple should not be joined in holy matrimony" and that I had been instructed by the parties to proceed with the ceremony.'

'My goodness, Reverend Jenkinson, I never realised that conducting a wedding ceremony could be so problematic.'

'Oh believe me it can be. That's not the first time something like that has happened to me. Christenings and funerals are far less likely to give trouble. Anyway I've taken up enough of your time so I'll be on my way. Goodbye for now and may God bless you.'

'Goodbye, Reverend Jenkinson and thank you for the wine.'

Wendy had been hovering in the hallway whilst I was talking to Reverend Jenkinson and she was naturally anxious to get into my surgery to familiarise herself with the layout. She mounted the stairs at great speed leaving me trailing way behind. Presumably Spencer had shown her the room when she came for her interview because she knew exactly where to go. She immediately started opening drawers and cupboards noting their contents.

'Hand instruments, forceps and surgical instruments, local anaesthetic, needles, cements, root canal instruments, white filling materials, rubber dams, burs' polishing strips and finishing stones' she recited, making a mental note of where things were stored. 'I've more or less got it,' she declared. 'It will take a little while before I'm completely used to it but I'm ready to start as soon as your first patient arrives.'

'That's incredible, Wendy. Can you really memorise the layout of the surgery that quickly?'

'Try me,' she said. 'Ask me to get something for you and we'll see if I can remember where it's kept.'

'Root canal sealer,' I said, thinking that this would really test her because some dentists might store it with the other cements whilst others might keep it with the root filling equipment. Quick as a flash she went to the cupboard housing the cements and pointed to the root canal sealer.

'That's fantastic, Wendy; I'm most impressed.'

'As I said, it will take a little while for me to be really efficient but I've a pretty good idea where things are kept now. Until recently I ran a dental nursing agency whereby dentists used to phone me and ask me to help out at short notice, when for example their nurse was ill, which meant that I was working in strange surgeries all the time so I had to learn to adapt quickly.'

As we were speaking, I was aware of heavy, clumping footsteps on the stairs and I looked up to see a tall, white-haired old man standing in the doorway. He was wearing baggy corduroy trousers, an old tweed jacket and a monocle and was carrying a highly polished walking stick. He had a pointed chin and a nose to match which twisted to the right as he struggled to retain his monocle in position.

'James Rutherford MA, at your service. You must be Mr Derwent.'

'Indeed I am, Mr Rutherford. Please come in and take a seat.'

'So you are my new dentist – a strange calling for one so young. I cannot understand why anyone would want to spend their entire life looking into people's mouths.'

'Someone has to do it,' I responded.

'*Let no-one honour me with tears, or bury me with lamentations. Why? Because I fly hither and thither, living in the mouths of men.*' He held up his right hand and articulated the words with the flourish and eloquence of a Shakespearian actor.

'Is that Shakespeare?' I ventured.

'No, my boy. Quintus Ennius – the father of Roman poetry. That's the trouble with scientists – and I would loosely describe you as a scientist – they tend to be very ignorant of the arts and literature in general, which is sad, because these are the things that really matter in life.'

'You may be right, Mr Rutherford, but when you've got toothache you need a quasi-scientist to get you out of trouble.'

'Ah, but *He that sleeps feels not the toothache.* Mercifully, I have no pain; well not much and I'm sure it can easily be put right.'

'If you'd like to sit down, I'll have a look.'

He moved from his position by the door and dropped heavily into my dental chair, reciting Shakespeare as he did so.

'*I saw young Harry rise from the ground like feather'd Mercury and vaulted with such ease into his seat.*

'I shall be most surprised if there's anything really wrong because it's no more than a few months since I graced these premises with my presence.'

'It's a bit longer than that, Mr Rutherford. It's over two years since your last check-up.'

'You greatly surprise me that two summers and winters have hurried by since I submitted to Mr Padginton's last rigorous assessment of my dental health. As you will discover for yourself one day, Mr Derwent, time passes at an ever increasing rate with advancing years, and in the wise words of W.B. Yeats – *The innocent and the beautiful have no enemy but time.*'

'Will you open your mouth and let me examine your teeth please, Mr Rutherford?'

'*Examinations are formidable even to the best prepared, for the greatest fool may ask more than the wisest man can answer.*'

'I don't think that refers to the sort of examination I'm talking about. I simply want to look at your teeth.'

'Examination is examination which, according to the Oxford English Dictionary, if I remember rightly, is defined as *the action of testing or judging by a standard.* Unless I am much mistaken, I imagine

86

that it is your intention to judge my dentition against an accepted standard and if it falls short of that standard in any way then you will no doubt wish to take remedial action to restore me to that standard.'

'That more or less sums it up. Now will you please open your mouth and let me see your teeth?'

'I am conscious of the fact that I am hindering your progress but we have only just met and I feel that it is only right and proper that we become better acquainted before I submit to the intimate and for me, humiliating experience of letting you inspect my dentition. After all, it is only natural to wish to consider carefully, the credentials of anyone who makes such a bold request, before allowing myself to be subjected to the indignity of such an entreaty.'

Wendy caught my eye and pointed to her watch to indicate that time was passing. I could see that my new nurse intended to make sure I worked efficiently but I was well aware that I had a busy morning ahead of me and I hadn't even got inside his mouth. I couldn't afford to run late with him or I would spend the rest of the morning trying to catch up. I was now beginning to lose patience.

'Mr Rutherford, I could understand your reluctance if I were intending to perform brain surgery on you, but as I merely want to look at your teeth will you please let me get on with it.'

He began to open his mouth. I'm not sure if it was to let me look at his teeth or whether he was about to say something else, but I didn't give him the option – I stuck my mirror on top of his tongue and eased it gently but swiftly into his mouth. I decided to keep it there because I felt sure that if I withdrew it, he would start talking again. I did my best to check his teeth but as Spencer had predicted they were completely covered in tartar so a proper examination was impossible. Nevertheless I looked all round before I released him. To begin with, he squirmed a little and made gurgling type noises as if trying to form words but I held firm. In the end, I think he realised his efforts were futile, and he gave up.

It was impossible to check for cavities because the tartar masked everything but it was clear that his gums were being severely irritated by the tartar and were in bad state. I placed my mirror and probe on the bracket table and wondered how I was going to approach this problem.

'Well my boy, what do you make of them? Eh? Eh? Not bad for an old timer are they? They've been around for a good many years now and have served me well.'

'Mr Padginton tells me you don't believe much in toothbrushing.'

'That's right – don't believe in it – never have, never will. My teeth have never given me much trouble so I saw no reason for meddling with them. I've only ever had toothache once in my life and that was when I was in a Japanese prisoner-of-war camp. I broke a piece off a tooth just before I was captured and didn't bother to get it sorted out. Well after a few weeks the blighter started to play me up. There was no medical help available, conditions were appalling and this damn tooth was driving me mad.

'One day I saw a Jap worker repairing a window and the idea struck me that if I could get hold of a bit of putty I could stop my tooth with it. That night after dark I crept out and waited until the guard's back was turned then crawled about two hundred yards on my belly dodging behind huts and piles of timber each time the guard looked my way.

'I waited for the right moment then leapt over to the window and dug my fingernails into the soft putty and dragged out as much as I could, then I jumped back under cover just before the guard turned. I don't mind telling you I was petrified. Then I had to crawl all the way back to my hut and all the time I risked being shot like a rabbit if the guard spotted me. My elbows were sore and bleeding by the time I got to my bed and amazingly, I'd forgotten about my toothache. I was so exhausted with excitement, fear and the sheer exertion of it all I just passed out still holding the lump of putty in my hand. When I woke up, the toothache was back with a vengeance so I plugged the hole with a bit of the putty. Actually I had enough to fill fifty teeth. I only needed a piece the size of a small pea and all that effort to get it.'

'It's an interesting story, Mr Rutherford,' I said thinking that interesting though it might be, I didn't really have time to stand there listening to it.

'I haven't finished yet. The putty didn't really help, in fact, to be honest, it was worse for a couple of days then the pain went away. Didn't taste too good either. Soon after that my face swelled up, then it went down, then it swelled up again. It was like that – up and down all the time I was in the prison camp. I had the tooth extracted soon after I got back to England after the war and do you know there was still some putty in there? I reckon I must have made a pretty good job of stopping it.'

'Remarkable,' I admitted as Wendy pointed to her watch again.

'That's the only time I've ever had trouble with my teeth and that's why I thought it best to leave them alone and not involve myself with all that tooth brushing business. I came here today because this one here,' pointing to an upper canine, 'the one I use for holding my pipe has become a bit shaky. It niggles a bit from time to time – not really toothache – nothing really. I thought I'd get you to stop it for me. I wouldn't have bothered if I could hold my pipe at the other side but somehow it doesn't feel right that way and in any case I've got a bit of arthritis in this elbow which makes it difficult to get this hand up to my face.'

'I'm afraid stopping it won't help,' I replied feebly.

'What do you mean, won't help? Of course it will help. Come along m'boy I want to get back to prune my roses; just get on with it, there's a good chap.'

'What I'm trying to say, Mr Rutherford, is that the problem with your tooth is not one that can be solved with a filling. There isn't a hole in it; it's aching and loose because of gum disease which has resulted from lack of proper tooth brushing.'

'Poppycock,' he grunted. 'Taken a hell of a long time to show itself.'

'I'm afraid it's true. Gum disease progresses very slowly in some people. In your case it's been going on for many years without causing any symptoms until now.'

'Well I go to the foot of our stairs,' he exclaimed still finding it hard to believe. 'What's the answer then? I don't want to lose any.'

'You may have to. If the gum disease has gone too far it may not be possible to save them. I shan't know until I've cleaned off all the tartar.'

'You've got to save them. I'm too old to start wearing plastic choppers. What do we have to do?'

'First of all you have to get a toothbrush and start using it at least twice a day, every day.'

'Isn't there any other way?'

'I'm afraid not. You won't really get any benefit until I've scaled all that tartar off and we'll need to make another appointment to do that but I want to try and get you into a tooth brushing routine right away. I don't suppose you own a toothbrush so I want you to buy one on your way home and start using it from today.'

He looked far from convinced and nodded half-heartedly without saying anything.

'Arrange another appointment as soon as possible. I shall probably need three quarters of an hour please, Wendy.'

Mr Rutherford had not paid much attention to her until now but as she removed his bib, he took hold of her hand and looked into her eyes.

'And always keep a hold of Nurse for fear of finding something worse.'

Wendy looked at him with an expression that suggested she thought he was completely mad and that she had not the slightest idea what he was talking about. 'She has great beauty,' he continued still holding her hand.

'Beauty is bought by judgment of the eye,
Not utter'd by base sale of chapmen's tongues.'

'That's Shakespeare, isn't it, Mr Rutherford?' I put forward, tentatively, desperately trying to remember where it came from and anxious to prove that I wasn't totally ignorant of all literature.

'You're right this time, Mr Derwent. I'd like to think it wasn't just a lucky guess. *'Love's Labour's Lost,* in fact.'

I heard the doorbell ring and knew that it was probably my next patient.

'Wendy, will you take Mr Rutherford downstairs and make him another appointment.'

Unfortunately, he wasn't yet ready to go.

'I need to speak to you about mother, Mr Derwent. She finds it very difficult to go out and about these days and I was wondering if it might be possible for you come and see her at home. I know it's a lot to ask of you, as you are clearly a very busy young man, but I make no stipulation as to when this should be. It can be entirely at your convenience. I am, however, conscious of the fact that this situation could change because her teeth have, sadly, been neglected for some considerable time.'

'Of course, I'll arrange to come and see her but you must appreciate that if she needs any treatment, it might not be possible to do it at home; it depends on what's needed. We might have to arrange transport to bring her to the surgery.'

'We shall face that obstacle if and when the need arises, Mr Derwent. Your offer to carry out a home visit is enough to set my mind at rest for the present. Shall I arrange a date with your delightful assistant?'

Mr Rutherford paused for a moment, reflecting upon what he had just said.

'I feel quite sure that a date with your lovely nurse is a pleasure I can only dream about,' he continued.

I ignored his ramblings and replied, 'we'll make arrangements for a home visit as soon as possible, Mr Rutherford. Go with Wendy and she'll arrange it for you.'

'Whilst I'm here, Mr Derwent, I need to talk to you about young Harold. He hasn't been at all well recently and unfortunately all his confidence appears to have deserted him. His teeth are in a very bad state and I think he's embarrassed about them. If we could smarten him up a bit, I'm sure it would help him to find his feet. I'm very concerned that he doesn't have any friends. He rarely goes anywhere these days though he did go to the Bath and West Show last year. We go there every year without fail; I think it's wonderful. Do you go, Mr Derwent?'

'No, I've never been.'

'You really should. How about you, nurse, do you go?'

'No,' Wendy replied.

'You don't know what you're missing – it's a most enjoyable day out. Anyway, I was telling you about young Harold. I'm most concerned about him because I have a suspicion that he might have started smoking and drinking in secret.'

'That must be a worry for you, Mr Rutherford. Harold's your son, I take it?'

'Indeed he is. My one and only.'

'Presumably he's able to come to the surgery?'

'Oh yes,' Mr Rutherford confirmed.

'Then there isn't a problem. You can make an appointment for him.'

'I will, Mr Derwent, but I want to warn you that he is a very sensitive young man and will need to be treated with the utmost care.'

'Don't worry, we'll look after him.'

Whilst we were speaking I was gradually advancing towards the door hoping he would retreat in the same direction. Wendy was well aware that we needed to hasten things along and took command of the situation.

'Come with me, Mr Rutherfford, and I'll arrange some appointments.'

She was polite but her authoritative tone of voice made it difficult for him to resist and she reinforced her request by holding out her hand to usher him along. It was expertly done and it made me realise that there was more to being a good dental nurse than simply being able to offer chair-side assistance. It was early days but I was already beginning to think that Spencer had done well in finding Wendy.

Mr Rutherford's departure left me feeling quite exhausted and I sat down to draw breath before dealing with my next patient. Spencer was wandering about and poked his nose into my surgery.

'Spoke about flying hither and thither and living in the mouths of men, did he?' Spencer queried.

'Amongst other things. I didn't do much dentistry but at least I feel that my knowledge of literature has increased and I've been given a good insight as to what life was like in a Japanese prisoner-of-war camp.'

'He used that particular quotation when he came to me for the first time. I wonder if it just came to mind or whether he spent hours searching for something appropriate.'

'I've no idea. But in addition to the quotations, I also had to listen to his story about how he stole some putty to stop his tooth whilst he was in a Japanese prisoner-of-war camp, then he talked about young Harold and his mother.'

As I said it, I realised that something didn't quite make sense. 'Mr Rutherford must be in his eighties, so his mother must be positively ancient. And if his son, Harold, is a young man, does Mr Rutherford have a young wife?'

Spencer provided the answer. '"Young Harold" is well into his sixties but has never married and has lived at home all his life, and "mother" is Mr Rutherford's wife – Harold's mother.'

'Now it makes sense. Apparently, "young Harold" has taken to smoking and drinking in secret.'

'Really,' Spencer retorted. 'I'm not surprised. Living with Mr Rutherford and "mother" would drive anyone to drink. I'm amazed he wasn't driven to it a long time ago. Perhaps he was, but Mr Rutherford didn't find out about it until recently. One thing's for sure, Harold won't be allowed to go out with any loose women.'

'Poor Harold. It sounds as though he's been stifled all his life.'

'I'm sure he has,' said Spencer. 'You saw what Rutherford was like. I don't envy you trying to treat "mother" either. She's as nutty as he is. As for "young Harold", I haven't had the pleasure of meeting him. He's made several appointments over the years, or should I say he's had appointments made for him, but he's never actually turned up so far. When the time comes, he can't face it, so be warned. You run the risk of having your time wasted!'

'Great,' I mumbled.

'What do you think of Wendy? Do you like her?'

'I'm most impressed with what I've seen so far, Spencer; it seems you may well have chosen wisely.'

CHAPTER FOURTEEN

The morning went quite smoothly after Mr Rutherford left. Fortunately, Wendy had persuaded him to leave my surgery before he had taken up too much time talking and I managed to get through to half past twelve without running late. I would have been on track for a one o'clock lunch had it not been for the fact that Mrs Jenson, who was the last patient of the morning, hadn't turned up.

'I thought I heard the doorbell. Are you sure Beryl didn't let her in?' I asked Wendy.

'Beryl didn't let her in: I checked.' Wendy replied. 'Is she often late?'

'No, never. I hope she's all right.' I looked at my watch. 'I'll give her another ten minutes; if she still hasn't shown up, I'll go to lunch.'

I actually waited a quarter of an hour, but the doorbell didn't ring during this time.

'It doesn't look as if she's coming,' I declared. 'I'm going to lunch now.'

'Okay, Justin. I'll see you this afternoon,' Wendy replied. 'I'm off to do some shopping.'

It was always a bit annoying when patients didn't turn up for their appointments but on this occasion I was more concerned than annoyed. Mrs Jenson was usually so reliable – in fact, I couldn't remember her ever failing an appointment before. I hoped she wasn't ill or had had an accident. I felt sure that even if she had become ill she would have done everything possible to let me know, so the fact that I hadn't heard from her was quite worrying. Perhaps she had simply forgotten – which could happen to anyone. I decided that if she didn't telephone whilst I was at lunch I would ask Wendy to contact her.

I took my coat from the office and ran down the stairs. As I passed the old waiting room, I noticed that the door was open, which was a bit strange, since the room was not being used now. Spencer had removed the sign from the door and I felt sure he would have closed it. Instinctively I went to shut it but something made me look into the room before I did so. Much to my surprise, I saw a very puzzled looking Mrs Jenson standing by the fireplace.

'Mrs Jenson,' I called out. 'What are you doing there?'

'I'm waiting for you, Mr Derwent. I had an appointment with you at twelve thirty.'

'I know. I thought you hadn't come. Didn't you realise that we'd moved the waiting room?'

'No. I thought it was a bit strange there wasn't any furniture in the room but I thought you must be decorating or something.'

I was amazed that Mrs Jenson had not attached greater importance to the fact that, not only was there no furniture, but there was not a single picture on the walls, and the rugs had been removed to reveal bare floorboards.

'We wouldn't have removed all the chairs even if we had been decorating because we wouldn't expect patients to wait standing up. And didn't you notice that the sign had been removed from the door?'

'I wasn't aware there was a sign on the door – I can't ever recall seeing it.'

'I was worried that you might be ill because I know you wouldn't fail an appointment without good reason.'

'No, I wouldn't, Mr Derwent. I suppose I've missed my appointment now?'

'I was leaving to go to lunch, but as you're here, I'll see you.'

'That's really kind of you, Mr Derwent, because it's quite a long bus ride for me to get here. I'm so pleased my journey won't have been in vain.'

'Come upstairs to the surgery and I'll try to catch Wendy before she leaves for lunch. She'll be surprised when she finds out you were here all the time.'

It took about twenty minutes to complete Mrs Jenson's treatment which meant that I had to cut short my lunch break in order to be ready for my first patient of the afternoon at two o'clock. Spencer didn't start his afternoon session until two thirty because of his habitual after-lunch sleep, and his first patient of the afternoon was one of the two female students he had told me about.

They arrived together, though I didn't see them because I was treating someone else at the time; then just after half past two, Beryl escorted one of them to Spencer's surgery. I happened to see her as she disappeared through his door and I felt sure that he had picked out the one he wanted to see and left me with the other one. She was strikingly dressed in a very fashionable, purple, wet-look coat which came well below her knees hiding the tops of some equally fashionable black boots. She had short, dark hair and the sort of smile, which, when it belonged to a patient, made Spencer think that dentistry wasn't such a bad job after all. A good deal of laughter emanated from his surgery over the next quarter of an hour and I felt sure that Spencer was thoroughly enjoying himself, albeit in an entirely professional way.

As soon as I was ready to see her friend, I sent Wendy downstairs to fetch her and whilst I was waiting, I could hear the laughter in Spencer's surgery intensifying – so much so that I couldn't resist going to find out what it was all about.

'I'm terribly sorry, Mr Padginton,' I heard the girl say through paroxysms of giggling, 'but I'm stuck to your chair.'

Apparently her wet-look coat had somehow adhered itself to the age-polished leather of Spencer's chair and, despite her efforts, she was unable to get up.'

'It looks as if I'm stuck with you then, my dear,' Spencer replied. 'Never mind, I'm sure we shall get on very well together.'

At first, I don't think Spencer believed that she really couldn't get out of his chair. However, when he saw how she was struggling to get up and that her coat was well and truly attached to the leather, he realised she wasn't joking.

'Allow me,' he said with a smile; and with obvious enjoyment, he put his arms round her and tried to lift her up. He succeeded in elevating her, though he achieved it by hoisting her out of her coat, which remained firmly glued to his chair.

The girl thought it was highly amusing and couldn't stop laughing whilst Spencer was savouring every moment of this golden opportunity to hold the delightful creature in his arms. Slowly and with some hesitation he deposited her on her feet and released her from his grip. He then set about peeling her coat off his chair. She was helpless to assist because she was still rolling about with laughter.

'I'm terribly sorry, Mr Padginton,' the girl chuckled, trying to compose herself. 'I had no idea my coat would stick to your chair like that – I should have taken it off before I sat down.'

'Don't worry about it, my dear; no harm done. Your coat looks all right; I don't think it's been damaged in any way.'

At that point, I left them to it because I heard Wendy talking to the other student who was being escorted into my surgery. I felt sure, knowing Spencer as I did, that he would have chosen the student he liked the look of best, and so I wasn't expecting her friend to be anything like as attractive.

To say that I wasn't disappointed would be a gross understatement. She was gorgeous! She wasn't as flamboyantly dressed as her friend but she was no less stylish, wearing a camel-coloured duffle coat over a dark green sweater, a checked midi skirt and brown leather boots. She had lovely long auburn hair and the clearest, most beautiful blue eyes I had ever seen.

'Thank you so much for seeing me, Mr Derwent. I'm registered with a dentist in Southampton where I'm at university, but I'm at home with my parents at the moment and I shan't be going back to Southampton for a few days. I've got a bit of a problem which is making it difficult for me to study, so I called in this morning to see if you or your colleague would give me some advice.'

We shook hands and I invited her to sit in my chair. I saw from the record card, which Wendy had prepared, that her name was Harriet Brooks.

'Well, Harriet , what sort of problem is it?'

'I keep on getting mouth ulcers. I just get rid of one, and another one crops up. It's been going on for a few weeks now, and they can be very painful.'

'And you've got one at the moment?'

'Yes, underneath my tongue at the left side.'

'May I see?'

She opened her mouth to reveal a very good set of teeth with hardly any fillings and extremely healthy gums, apart from a very red and inflamed area exactly where she had indicated.

'I can see that it's very sore.'

'It certainly is and I don't know what to do about it. Is it anything serious?'

'No. Not at all. It's a typical aphthous ulcer – very painful and unpleasant, but not serious.' I said reassuringly.

'I'm pleased about that. Is there anything you can do to get rid of it and also to prevent me from getting any more?'

'I'm afraid there's no complete cure. Some people just seem to be prone to them, whilst other people very rarely, if ever, get them. We don't really know what causes them. It has been suggested that certain foods can trigger them off – citrus fruits are often blamed. And it was thought a virus could be responsible, but no-one has been able to identify one, and that theory seems to have lost favour. It does appear, however, that they are linked to stress in some people. Students often get them at exam time. Do you think this could be a factor in your case?'

'Well, I shall soon be taking my finals, so I suppose it's possible that could have something to do with it. But is there nothing you can do to help?'

Harriet sounded quite despondent to think I might not be able do anything to alleviate her suffering. Fortunately, I was able to offer her some hope.

'Although there's no actual cure, we've found that the use of a strong antiseptic mouthwash usually helps quite considerably. It probably works simply by preventing the ulcers from becoming infected and this makes them heal more quickly. I'll give you a prescription for something which tastes fowl, but is usually very effective if you use it morning and night. It should take the soreness away quite quickly. I have to tell you, though, it's very strong and I'm afraid it will affect your ability to taste your food.'

'I don't mind that if it works. As a student, my diet isn't very exciting – beans on toast mostly, so being unable to taste isn't going to matter very much.'

I wrote the prescription and handed it to her.

'Thank you so much for seeing me, Mr Derwent. I feel much better now that I know it isn't serious. I was worried it might be mouth cancer or something terrible. You have reassured me. How much do I owe you?'

'You don't owe me anything, Harriet. It was my pleasure to see you. I hope I've been able to help you and good luck with your finals. What are you studying?'

'Psychology.'

'Really? That's an interesting subject.'

'Yes, I find it fascinating. I'm very interested in people. I love to study them: to see how they behave and to find out what motivates them.'

'Then it sounds as if psychology is an ideal subject for you.'

'Yes, I think it is. I shall just be glad when I've got my finals out of the way.'

'I'm sure you'll sail through without any difficulty.'

'I don't know about that but thank you once again for your help, Mr Derwent.'

After Harriet had left, Wendy turned to me with a cheeky smile. 'You liked her didn't you, Justin?'

'She certainly made a very pleasant change from the old ladies with their dentures.'

'I think there was more to it than that.'

'I thought she was a very nice girl.'

'I could tell you liked her. It's a pity she's already got a dentist and that she's at university in Southampton.'

CHAPTER FIFTEEN

I was late getting home from work that day. The afternoon had gone smoothly enough until about four o'clock and then I started to run late. There was no particular reason for it – sometimes it just happens.

I was unlocking the door to my cottage after an uneventful drive home, when I heard the phone ringing inside. It always seemed to ring just after I got in the door – usually whilst I was making a cup of tea. Tonight I hadn't got that far, it started when I was still outside. I thought it might be Sarah but it wasn't; it was Richard Darcy.

'Hello, Justin. How are you?'

'Fine, thank you, Richard. How are you?'

'I'm well. I'm phoning to see if you're free this evening because I'm thinking of going to a nightclub, called The Twilight Club, and I wondered if you wanted to come with me.'

'Here we go again,' I said to myself. 'The never-ending hunt for women.'

'It's at Halfington,' Richard continued. 'Apparently it opened nearly two years ago but I only heard about it yesterday. I thought it might be worth a try. Would you like to go?'

I wasn't particularly enthusiastic, I found nightclubs to be dark, hot, smoky and very noisy and I didn't think that going there to try to pick up girls was the best way to meet that 'special someone', which presumably was the aim of the exercise. However, I didn't want to disappoint Richard and I didn't have any other plans.

'Yes, all right. What time are you going?'

'I'll call for you at eight. I'll drive.'

'See you later then,' I replied, thinking that if he came to collect me, at least I wouldn't have to witness his obsessional behaviour when he checked that everything electrical was switched off and unplugged before leaving his house. I guessed that he didn't want to go in my car because it only had two seats, which would present a problem if we picked up any girls.

He arrived at five past eight and soon we were on our way to Halfington.

'Have you had a good day?' he began the conversation.

'Not too bad. The highlight of it was early this afternoon when I had a young psychology student come to see me. I thought she was quite lovely.'

'Did you ask her out?'

No, of course not. She came as a patient. I couldn't ask her out.'

'Why ever not?'

'Because it would have amounted to an abuse of our professional relationship.'

'Stuff that! If you meet someone you like the look of, you can't afford to miss the opportunity to get to know her better. I can't see what the problem is. She's hardly likely to report you just for inviting her out for a drink. If she fancies you, she'll be pleased to accept, and if she doesn't, she only has to refuse. In any event, she'll probably be flattered that you asked her.'

'Well, I didn't.'

'Will you be seeing her again?'

'It's most unlikely. She's at university in Southampton, and has a dentist there. She's visiting her parents at the moment, who live somewhere around here, and she came to see me because she had a slight dental problem. I think I've sorted it out for her so it's unlikely that she'll come back to see me again.'

'That's a great pity and it sounds like a missed opportunity to me. Are you still seeing Sarah Hanson?'

'Yes. I went out with her yesterday but it was a bit of a disaster because we got stuck in a flood. I tried to drive through some water on the road, which turned out to be quite deep and my car conked out. Fortunately, a farmer towed us out and managed to get it going again, but it put an end to our plans to go for a walk by the sea at Westport. In any case, the weather was atrocious. We went back to her house and spent the rest of the day with her mother and her dogs for company.'

'How exciting,' Richard scoffed. 'Are you still keen on her?'

'I like her, but there were two things she said yesterday that gave me some cause for concern. First, she tried to make me promise not to see you again because she thinks you're a bad influence.'

Richard guffawed. 'I'm flattered that she thinks I have such sway. The fact that you're here with me now suggests that you weren't prepared to make that promise.'

'You're right; I wasn't.'

'What did she say when you refused?'

'I didn't make a big issue of it and I didn't actually refuse outright. I just didn't make any promises and I quickly changed the subject.'

'So you dodged the issue, really?'

'Yes, I suppose I did.'

'To my mind, it augurs badly for the future. Before you know it, you'll be completely under her thumb unless you stamp on it immediately. To be perfectly honest, if I were you, I'd get rid of her before you get in any deeper.'

'It sounds a bit ruthless.'

'Believe me, as a solicitor with considerable experience of divorce cases, I can tell you that it's frequently necessary to be ruthless where women are concerned.'

'That's a pretty cynical attitude.'

'Perhaps it is, but I've seen far too many marriages break down because the early warning signs were ignored by one of the parties. It isn't always the woman at fault; though I have to say that, in my experience: it usually is.'

'Isn't it often the man who goes off with someone else?'

'It can be, but you have to ask yourself what makes him do it. In many cases he's driven to it.'

'You seem to have a poor opinion of women in general. Is that why you never seem to form a lasting relationship?'

Richard appeared to be rather taken aback by my question. For a moment I thought I might have offended him.

'It's true that I'm extremely cautious,' he answered.

'Perhaps you're too cautious. Nobody's perfect and unless you're prepared to accept some shortcomings, you'll never find a partner.'

'You could be right but I'm not prepared to take any risks with my future. If you choose the wrong woman it can be very difficult, expensive, and messy to get rid of her.'

'How did you get on with Denise?'

'Denise? Oh yes; the nurse from the hospital. I only saw her once. She failed the Mahler test, I'm afraid. I took her back to my place and played her Mahler's Fourth. She said she hated it – told me she doesn't like any classical music; she likes Elton John and Neil Diamond. Neil Diamond! – I ask you! Pretty as she is, I couldn't see much future there. Anyway, going back to Sarah Hanson, what else did she say to you that gave you cause for concern? Was that about me as well?'

'No, it wasn't about you. She wants me to go on a weekend course with her to learn how to parachute jump.'

Richard's reaction was complete shock and horror, and his car swerved as the full impact of Sarah's ambition hit him.

'Jesus Christ! You mean that she wants you to jump out of a plane?'

'Exactly that. You spend the weekend learning how to do it and the climax comes on the Sunday afternoon when they take you up and you jump out.'

'Hell's bells! There's no way on earth I would even think about doing that. You wouldn't get me in a plane in the first place, not even a Jumbo jet, let alone expect me to jump out of the bloody thing. You'd have to be mental to even contemplate it. The woman must be stark raving mad to want to do it. You're not going to, are you?'

'I'm not keen on the idea but I haven't actually told her yet that I won't do it.'

'Not keen on the idea? Not keen on the idea? You need your head examined if you have anything to do with it. Get out of the relationship whilst you're still in one piece. The woman's obviously completely balmy. If you stay with her, before you know it she'll have you doing all sorts of ridiculous things like running marathons, trying to swim the channel, climbing mountains, potholing or deep sea diving.'

'I don't think so. It's just that she's always wanted to parachute jump but doesn't want to do it on her own, so she's asked me to go with her. She thinks it would be romantic to jump out of the plane holding hands.'

'It won't be very romantic when she discovers, on reaching the ground – *if* you get down in one piece – that you've wet yourself, or worse. I've never heard anything so ridiculous in my life. For God's sake get rid of the woman before she does you serious harm.'

Richard had made his thoughts on the subject abundantly clear and there seemed little point in discussing it further. In any case, we were about to arrive at the Twilight Club and Richard's thoughts turned to finding a suitable place to park his precious car.

The Club was situated in a narrow street just off the main road through the town and Richard was very reluctant to leave his car there for fear of someone scratching or denting it as they tried to squeeze past.

'I think I'll park round the corner on the main road,' he announced, putting the car into gear. The main road was quite wide and there were plenty of places to park but Richard was very choosy.

'I want to park under a street light because there's less chance of someone breaking in to it if it's well lit.'

'There's a space by that street light over there,' I suggested, pointing to a spot some thirty yards down the road.

'I saw that one,' Richard rejoined, 'but I'm not parking in front of a Transit Van. In my experience, Transit drivers are irresponsible idiots who don't have an ounce of respect for anyone else on the road — and they drive like lunatics. If I park there I'm likely to get my rear bumper ripped off if he leaves before I do.'

'You can't say that about all Transit drivers, Richard.'

'I've never met a sensible one yet. Anyway, I'm not prepared to risk it — I'll find somewhere else to park.'

After much driving up and down the main road, Richard spotted a car about to pull out from a space immediately under a streetlight. He waited impatiently for the driver to move off and then slowly and deliberately manoeuvred into position. When he had satisfied himself that he was equidistant from the cars in front and behind and that he was as close to the kerb as possible without actually scrubbing his tyres against it, he switched off his engine. He then went through his usual ritual of checking each door and the boot in turn to ensure that everything was secure. Only when he had repeated this procedure three times was he happy to leave the car.

It took less than five minutes to walk to the Twilight Club and as we approached the entrance, it became apparent that the building in which the Club was situated was in a poor state of repair. The windows were boarded on the inside to stop anyone from looking in and many of the panes of glass were broken. The wooden frames were all badly in need of paint and some of them were actually rotten. There was a flight of four stone steps leading to double doors which were invitingly wedged open with a couple of bricks. The doorman, or perhaps to be more accurate, the bouncer, greeted us as we stepped inside.

'Welcome to the Twilight Club, gentlemen. Have you been here before?'

'No, this is our first time,' Richard replied.

'In that case, you'll need to complete a simple registration form and as it's your first visit, you're entitled to a fifty percent discount off the usual entry fee by way of an introductory offer.' He pointed towards another door. 'The receptionist is through there on the left. She'll deal with your registration.'

I filled in the form, which merely asked for a name, an address, date of birth, and a telephone number, but I could see that Richard was distinctly uneasy about providing the information. I think it flickered across his mind to use a fictitious name and address but after a moment's pause he scribbled down his details in such a way that his writing was virtually illegible and he handed the form to the receptionist. She glanced at it and placed it on one side without comment except to say, 'That will be four pounds fifty each.'

'I thought we were supposed to be getting a fifty per cent discount?' queried Richard.

'Yes. That's right,' she confirmed. 'It's normally nine pounds unless you buy a season ticket. It works out much cheaper if you do.'

'No thanks,' said Richard, grudgingly handing over a ten pound note. 'Put the change in the charity box.'

The receptionist looked a little taken aback but before she was able to explain that they didn't have a charity box, Richard pointed to another pair of double doors and said 'I take it we go through there?'

She nodded.

The doors had excellent sound deadening properties because, when they were closed, the music within was barely audible but as soon as we opened them our ears were assaulted by strains of *Dancing Queen* by Abba at tremendous volume. The doors were also effective in enclosing an eye-watering level of cigarette smoke which billowed forth, the moment it was allowed to escape.

CHAPTER SIXTEEN

There was no ambient lighting in the room and all the illumination was provided by pulsating, flashing and rotating light sources which created an effect likely to trigger off an epileptic attack in anyone the slightest bit susceptible. Richard and I inched our way forward very slowly and cautiously, because the sudden bombardment of all our senses at the same instant caused total confusion and for a while, we felt completely disorientated. We peered into the gloom trying to penetrate the smog in order to make sense of what was going on. At first, all we could be sure of was that there were quite a lot of people there, though not many of them were dancing.

Very slowly our eyes adjusted to the lighting conditions and the surroundings became somewhat less muddled. I was able to ascertain that there were tables all around the outside of the room and more of them at one end, where the bar was situated. The other end was dominated by an enormous bank of loudspeakers which were responsible for the ear-splitting volume of the music emanating from that area. Much of the floor in front of the speakers was uncluttered to allow dancing and perched up on a platform centrally between the speakers and slightly behind the line of them, was the disc jockey.

We stood for some minutes surveying the room. Neither of us spoke. We would have had to shout to make ourselves heard and we both accepted that normal conversation would be nearly impossible and extremely tiring, so we independently resolved to use speech sparingly. The thought crossed my mind that if we went over to the bar, the music might not be quite so loud over there, and I was about to suggest this to Richard when I became aware of a man walking towards us. As he got nearer, I realised I had seen him somewhere before, though at first, I was unable to remember where. Richard provided the answer.

'Oh God, it's the halfwit with the ear-ring and trainers who goes to the Lord Nelson nearly every evening.'

'Oh yes,' I replied. 'I remember seeing him the last time we went there together. You weren't very complimentary about him on that occasion.'

'Well look at him. Would you grant him bail? He's a complete moron.'

The man, who was wearing a white T-shirt bearing the words *Try Me* and flared blue jeans, swaggered up to Richard and began to speak to him.

'Hi, Dick. Fancy seeing you here.'

Richard violently objected to his name being abbreviated in this way particularly by someone for whom he felt utter contempt, and he retorted with venom.

'There may be a lot of dicks here tonight; but I'm not one of them.' He turned and walked away from the man leaving him in no doubt that their conversation was over.

'You were a bit hard on him, weren't you, Richard? The poor chap was trying to be friendly.'

'He's an absolute jerk and I've never forgiven him for trying to persuade me to put in a good word for him with the police in order to get him off a speeding fine. He picked the wrong person when he asked me. I took it as an insult that he thought I would be prepared even to consider such a thing. If it had been up to me I'd have added the charge of "attempting to pervert the course of justice" to the speeding offence. I've no time for him. Anyway, let's get a drink.'

As we walked over to the bar, another, somewhat older man approached. He was wearing an open-necked red shirt and a pair of blue jeans and had a gold medallion nestling in the abundant growth of hair on his chest. I recognized him also as someone I had seen in the Lord Nelson. For some reason, Richard seemed slightly less hostile to this man and was the first to speak.

'Hello, Tony. Fancy seeing you here.'

'Good evening, Richard. Welcome to Grab a Granny. I've not seen you here before.'

'Grab a Granny? What's that?'

'It's what we call this place. If you look at the women here you'll see why. Most of them are drawing the old-age pension.'

Richard looked stunned. 'We've only just arrived. We haven't had time to look round yet, but if the women are as bad as that, why do you come?'

'It's just another place to hang out, and you just never know, there might be someone here worth a second glance one of these days. Occasionally you get someone who's a bit younger, and we live in hope.'

'Who's we?' Richard demanded, still reluctant to accept that the Club held such little promise, particularly after paying four pounds fifty to get in.

'Jim, Dave, Dino, Steve, Pedro and Jack – the usual gang'

'I saw that stupid Jim. Are all of you here?'

'Sure are,' Tony confirmed, 'we've got season tickets. Works out much cheaper that way.'

'Bloody hell,' Richard groaned and walked away from Tony in utter disgust.

'That lot bloody well haunt me. Every time I go into the Lord Nelson they seem to be there, in fact they seem to follow me around. If I decide to go somewhere else for a change, nine times out of ten they'll turn up there. I don't seem to be able to shake them off.'

'So they do the rounds like you, looking for women?'

'They certainly do the rounds but I've yet to see any of them pick up a woman.'

'But you see them as competition?'

Richard burst out laughing. 'Don't be ridiculous, Justin. You saw them – well two of them. Do you honestly think that any woman in her right mind is going to be interested in imbeciles like that? I've seen more respectable individuals in the dock charged with armed robbery.'

'I honestly don't know what women are interested in. I expect there are some women who might be attracted to them. If most of the women here are pensioners they might be willing to accept anything on offer.'

'Well, Justin, I can assure you I'm not interested in pensioners, Tony and his cronies are welcome to them. It sounds as though this place is a dead loss but I think we should have a good look round and check it out for ourselves. It could be that Tony was just spinning us a yarn because he sees us as competition. Perhaps he thought that if he told us it was no good, we'd leave.'

We pushed our way through the groups of people standing and those sitting at tables and after waiting several minutes for the over-worked barman to get around to serving us, Richard ordered a gin and tonic for himself and a pint of lager for me.

'That will be four pounds, please, sir.'

'What?' Richard exclaimed. 'That's extortionate.'

'I'm sorry, sir, but that's the cost. There's a list of bar prices over there.'

'I'll pay,' I offered, handing over the money to avoid further confrontation with the barman who was already stressed by the sheer number of people demanding attention. Richard merely grunted and said nothing. We took our drinks and moved away.

'My eyes have adjusted to the lighting now,' said Richard. 'Let's have a good look around to see what's on offer.'

'What about the woman in the black sweater over there. She looks quite nice,' I suggested.

'Do me a favour,' Richard replied harshly. 'Have you seen her legs? They look as though they've been fitted on upside down.'

He set off to survey the entire room systematically as if conducting a military reconnaissance exercise. I followed behind him as he started at the end of the room by the bar and worked his way along the line of tables scanning the faces of everyone sitting and standing. It was a slow and methodical search and the first phase of it turned out to be fruitless.

'It appears that Tony was telling the truth. The average age of the women I've seen so far is about seventy,' groaned Richard in despair.

We were now quite close to the disc jockey's loudspeakers and before I could answer, the voice of Gloria Gaynor singing *Never Can Say Goodbye* at an unbelievable volume totally crushed any chance of my being heard so I kept quiet. Richard rested his back against the wall and diverted his scrutiny to the other side of the room. He took a short sip of his gin and tonic and sighed looking quite deflated.

I leaned against the wall beside him and as I looked across the dance floor I caught sight of someone who I thought looked vaguely familiar. It was an elderly woman, heavily made up with bright red lipstick, powdered cheeks and wearing what looked like a dark blond wig. I was sure I recognized her face but I was unable to think where or when I'd seen her before and I couldn't help staring as I strived to identify her. Suddenly she caught my gaze and smiled back at me which confirmed that I did know her from somewhere. Perhaps she was a patient. I saw so many and it was often difficult to put a name to a face. She started to walk over towards me and then it hit me who she was.

'Oh my God,' I called out. 'It's Sarah's mother.'

For a moment, Richard didn't understand what I was saying. 'Sarah's mother? What are you talking about?'

When she came up to me and spoke, the situation gradually became clear to him.

'Hello, Justin,' she said. 'What are you doing here?'

I felt like putting the same question to her but I decided against it. 'My friend Richard asked me to come with him. We haven't been here before. Do you come here often?'

'Not often. I've been here a couple of times before but it isn't really my scene. I too, am here with a friend – that's her over there.'

The one in the blue dress, chatting to the two men?'

'Yes, that's her.'

'Did you meet the men here or did they come with you?'

It occurred to me that she might think my question rather impertinent and I'm not sure why I asked it, as it was none of my business. I suppose it was borne out of my own feelings of awkwardness about meeting her there. She would undoubtedly tell Sarah, who would not be too pleased to think I was out on the town, with Richard Darcy of all people, in a nightclub. It definitely suggested that I was not ready to make any sort of serious commitment to her, and whilst this might be true, I didn't particularly want the fact to be pushed down Sarah's throat.

'They didn't come with us but we've seen them here before so they aren't complete strangers,' she explained.

It was clear that she too felt a little uneasy. I don't suppose she wanted her daughter's boyfriend to think she was out looking for men any more than I wanted her to go back and tell Sarah I was there looking for women.

'Sarah's at home on her own this evening, Justin.'

I wasn't sure if she told me this to make me feel guilty or whether it was simply because she was finding it difficult to think of something to say to me.

'Is she?' I replied. 'I'll phone her.'

'She'll like that. Anyway it was nice to see you but I should go back to my friends now. I hope I shall see you again soon.'

'Yes. Have a pleasant evening, Mrs. Hanson. Goodbye.'

'And you, Justin, Goodbye.'

'The words "mutton" and "lamb" spring to mind,' said Richard somewhat uncharitably as soon as she was far enough away not to be able to hear.

'It's a bit sad, really,' I suggested. 'The poor woman lost her husband some years ago and life must get a bit lonely for her at times. Why shouldn't she come to somewhere like this in the hope of meeting a companion? Why should it be less acceptable for her than for you and I?'

'Good point, Justin. It's just that there seems to be something slightly disgusting about older people going out to pick up members of the opposite sex.'

'You might still be doing it yourself when you're older unless you're prepared to be a bit less fussy about who you form a long-term relationship with. In any case, she might just be here to try to make friends – she's not necessarily hoping to pick up men.'

'Well, looking around, it seems that most of the people here are her age; we're the odd ones out. I don't think this is the right place for us and although it grieves me to leave so soon, having paid four pounds fifty to get in, I think we should cut our losses and adjourn. We might do better at Fraser's Wine Bar.'

CHAPTER SEVENTEEN

.

'My goodness you look rough this morning,' was the greeting I received from Wendy as I slumped into the chair at my desk.

'A night out with Richard Darcy,' I grunted. 'Any chance of some coffee?'

'I'll go and make you some. Black and strong is called for I would imagine.'

'What are we doing this morning? I hope it isn't anything too demanding.'

'You're in luck actually,' said Wendy comfortingly, 'because Mr and Mrs Alexander who had an hour and half between them have cancelled as they've both gone down with some sort of horrible stomach bug. Mr Alexander said he would be prepared to battle on and keep his appointment as he didn't want to waste your time but Mrs Alexander is so bad she can't get out of bed. I didn't think you'd want to see him so I told him to stay at home and look after his wife. I've rebooked them.'

'Thank God for that. It was very noble of him to offer to keep his appointment but I feel bad enough already without a stomach bug to add to my misery. Does that mean I can sit and nurse my aching head for the first part of the morning?'

'Not quite. Mrs Newman telephoned just after I spoke to Mr Alexander and said she wanted to talk to you about something. I don't think she's in trouble but as you had some spare time I told her to come here at nine-thirty.'

Wendy's coffee worked its magic and by the time Mrs Newman arrived I was beginning to feel much better.

'Come in and sit down, Mrs Newman. What can I do for you?'

'I hope you won't laugh at me and think I'm being silly, Mr Derwent, but there's something I want to discuss with you. It's been on my mind for some time now but I haven't been able to pluck up enough courage to mention it. Finally, I decided I must act before it's too late. Provided you think it's possible of course.'

'I'm intrigued, Mrs Newman. I'll help if I can.'

Mrs Newman rummaged in the old shopping bag she was carrying and produced a very glossy magazine on the cover of which was the photograph of an undeniably glamorous, though to my mind somewhat toothy model. 'I want my teeth to look like that,' she exclaimed.

Her request came as a great surprise to me because my candid opinion was that she and the model had absolutely nothing in common. Mrs Newman had never paid much attention to her appearance. Her clothes were drab, she hardly wore any make-up and I imagined that visiting the hairdresser was a fairly infrequent event. Her teeth were healthy and even, but with some spacing and were very small to the point where they hardly showed at all, even on the rare occasions that she smiled. My first reaction was that teeth like those displayed by the model would not have suited her and I tried as tactfully as possible to convince her accordingly.

'I've thought long and hard about it, Mr Derwent, and my mind is made up. Please help me if you can.'

'It's true that your teeth don't show very much and it might be an improvement if we make them slightly bigger and close up the spaces between them but we need to be very careful as it could look really awful if we overdo it.'

'But they're so tiny at present. It doesn't look as if I've got any teeth. I'd so like to look like that.' She looked wistfully at the magazine she was clutching.

'I'll tell you what we can do this morning. As your teeth are spaced, I can slip some temporary plastic crowns over them, then we can get some idea how you'd look and it will also tell us by how much we could enlarge them.'

It took only a few minutes to place what I thought were sensibly sized plastic crowns over Mrs Newman's upper front teeth and I had to admit that closing the spaces was a distinct improvement. Wendy handed her a mirror. 'There aren't fixed so you'll need to be careful that they don't fall off but it's just to give you some idea how they'd look.'

'It's certainly better,' Mrs Newman declared. She studied her appearance for some moments then looked at the photograph on the magazine. 'But they need to be bigger, much bigger; they still don't show enough.'

'Are you sure, Mrs Newman? These crowns are quite a lot bigger than your teeth and as I said earlier, it can look awful if it's overdone.'

'I know what I want, Mr Derwent, and these aren't big enough.'

I sighed, as I firmly believed that the crowns I had fitted were already quite large and that to go any further would not look sensible but Mrs Newman seemed to have given the matter considerable thought and after all, she had to be satisfied.

'So how much bigger would you want them? Can you show me?'

'About half as long again, I would say.'

Wendy gave me a look of mild incredulity and smiled. I wondered how I could convince Mrs Newman that perhaps she was slightly misguided.

'That's an awful lot and I think that if we made them as long as that you wouldn't like them.' I replied, but I was becoming increasingly aware that it was going to be difficult to change her views. 'I don't have any other suitable temporary crowns we could try so what I'll do is take an impression of your teeth now and I'll get the technician to make up some plastic crowns just to see how they look. If and when we've established exactly how big you want them and we're sure they'll look sensible, we'll then think about going ahead with some permanent crowns. How does that sound?'

'That sounds a good idea, Mr Derwent, but you won't fit the permanent crowns until I'm sure they're going to be big enough, will you?'

'Of course not; you have to be one hundred percent happy before I do anything.'

'Thank you so much, Mr Derwent, I do want this treatment very badly and it will change my life if I can get it done.'

After Mrs Newman had left, Wendy paused from wrapping up the impression to send to the technician and looked at me thoughtfully. 'Mrs Newman seems to have a very clear idea what she wants, do you think her teeth will look ridiculous if we make them as big as she is requesting?'

'To be perfectly honest, yes I do. I've seen this sort of thing many times with dentures. A patient comes in with a denture saying they don't like it because the teeth don't show enough or they show too much. We wax up a new one and get them to look at it and then they start wanting alterations made. By the time we've finished we usually end up with something that is very similar to the one they've already got. It seems they think they want to change things but in truth they don't really want to look any different.'

'I'm not sure that's the case with Mrs Newman. I think her mind is well and truly made up that she wants bigger teeth.'

'You could be right. What I'm worried about is that she'll say the temporary crowns look all right so then we go ahead with the permanent ones making them the same size and she goes away happy, that is until her friends, surprised at the transformation, say "what the hell have you had done to your teeth; they look awful". A month later she'll be back saying she wants the crowns removed because she doesn't like them. Patients have also got very short memories. She'll swear it was my idea to make them really big; she'll say she wanted them much smaller but I persuaded her that they'd look better if they showed more. And as it was my fault, she'll want her money back.'

'You're beginning to develop a cynical streak in your old age, Justin. Are you sure general practice is good for you?'

CHAPTER EIGHTEEN

I thought it would only be a matter of time before Sarah telephoned and I wasn't looking forward to speaking to her because I knew she would be annoyed and upset that I had gone out with Richard Darcy. I felt sure her mother would have told her she saw us at the Twilight Club and the fact that I had met up with him the very next day after she had requested me not to, would only make things worse in her eyes. The final straw was that we had gone to a nightclub of all places, which would suggest to her I was up to no good.

I didn't have long to wait before the phone rang. I had driven home from work under rapidly-gathering storm clouds and thunder was rumbling in the distance. It had been raining on and off for the last three days and it looked as though the unsettled weather was set to continue into the night. The telephone call came after I'd been in my cottage for about ten minutes. I felt sure it would be Sarah ringing, and I wasn't wrong.

'Hello, Justin.'

'Hello, Sarah. How are you?'

'I'm not very happy, Justin. Are you surprised?'

'There's really no reason for you to be unhappy.'

'You broke your promise to me.'

'What promise is that, Sarah?'

'You promised me you wouldn't go out with Richard Darcy.'

'I didn't promise.'

'Yes, you did.'

'No I didn't. I know you wanted me to, but I wasn't prepared to make that promise so I changed the subject. I'm quite certain I didn't promise anything.'

'You led me to believe you were prepared to give up seeing him.'

'You made that assumption, but I can assure you I was most careful not to make any promises. I do remember saying to you that I value his friendship even though he might have some ways and opinions I don't' necessarily agree with.'

'So you aren't prepared to stop seeing him?'

'No, I'm not. But I don't see why you should have a problem with that.'

'I was very upset that you went to a nightclub. You were obviously looking for girls. After all, don't people usually go to nightclubs in order to meet members of the opposite sex?'

'Ask your mother.'

As soon as I said it, I felt a bit guilty. How Sarah's mother chose to spend her evenings was none of my business and I sensed that Sarah was slightly embarrassed.

'She goes there very occasionally with a friend just for a night out. She's not looking for men.'

'If you believe she's not looking for men, why don't you believe me when I say I'm not looking for women?'

'Did you meet any girls last night?'

'You must be joking. Even if we'd been looking, we weren't likely to find any at Grab a Granny.'

'At what?'

'Grab a Granny. Apparently that's what people call the Twilight Club.'

'Is it? I've not heard that before.'

'Well they do, and I can understand why.' I was about to say that it is frequented by old-age pensioners but because of her mother, I said. 'It seems to be popular with older people.'

'Will you be going again?'

'I very much doubt it; I don't really like nightclubs. I only went there because Richard wanted to go but I don't think he was very impressed. For a start, it's very expensive unless you buy a season ticket and, as I said, it seems to be a meeting place for older people.'

The anger had now gone out of Sarah's voice and she sounded more contrite.

'You didn't go there to pick up girls did you, Justin?'

'Of course not, Sarah; it isn't my style to do that. Richard wanted to go, and I suppose he was hoping to meet someone, but I just went with him. If I'm honest, I enjoy watching him in action when he meets someone he likes the look of and then sets about chatting them up. Personally, I don't think that's the best way to meet people and in any case, I'm no good at chatting up.'

'You're not envious of him are you?'

'No. Not in the slightest. I find him interesting and amusing but I wouldn't want to be like him.'

'I'm pleased about that, Justin. I'm sorry I got upset but I couldn't bear to think you were out looking for girls. Can I see you again?'

'Yes of course, Sarah. How about Saturday evening?'

'Saturday's a long way off. Can't I see you before then?'

'I'm sorry but I've a lot on this week.'

I didn't actually have any other plans for the week but I felt I needed a bit of breathing space and I still felt uneasy about Sarah trying to control my life.

'Are you going out with Richard again this week?' she asked hesitantly.

'I haven't arranged to see him. We only go out together occasionally – it isn't a regular thing.'

'All right then, Saturday.'

'I'll pick you up at seven.'

'I'll be ready. Has your car recovered from the soaking it suffered?'

'It's drying out slowly. The engine seems to have survived though, which is the main thing.'

'I'll see you on Saturday then, Justin.'

'Yes, at seven. Goodbye, Sarah.'

'Goodbye, Justin.'

I put down the phone and my attention turned towards eating. I hadn't had much lunch and I was now extremely hungry. As usual, however, an inspection of the refrigerator and the kitchen cupboards revealed that I had nothing in store which would even begin to satisfy my appetite. There seemed no alternative but to go shopping – an activity I found   tedious at the best of times but particularly so when tired and hungry after a hard day's work. There was a useful mini-supermarket in the square at Luccombury, very close to the practice, and it would have been sensible if I'd called in there after work. Time and time again I'd tried to get into the habit of doing this in an attempt to introduce some organization into my life but so far I had failed. Cursing my lack of planning I jumped into my car and drove back into the town. The thunder appeared to be getting closer and lightning was dancing over the distant hills but so far it still wasn't raining.

One advantage of shopping at that time in the evening was that the shops were usually quiet. Movement around the store was quick and unimpeded and soon I had a basket filled with bread, cheese, fruit, vegetables, fish and a bottle of wine. It had taken me less than twenty minutes since leaving my cottage and as I headed for the checkout, I felt confident that the entire operation would be completed and I would be back at home in a little over half an hour.

As I approached the checkout, my spirits were lifted by the sight of an attractive, young, female face apparently smiling in my direction. The face was familiar and I immediately recognised it as belonging to Harriet Brooks – the psychology student who came to see me as a patient yesterday.

'Hello, Mr Derwent. I didn't expect to see you here.'

'Shopping isn't my favourite pastime but I'm afraid it's unavoidable if you want to eat.'

'I don't like shopping either but my mother said she needed to buy some food and she wanted me to come with her. Unfortunately, it started thundering and she's terrified of it.'

'So where is she now?' I enquired, as there was no sign of anyone else near the checkout.'

Harriet laughed mischievously and as she did so her eyes sparkled and her face lit up in a devastatingly alluring way. 'She's in the car hiding under a travel rug, which is what she always does if she's out and it starts to thunder. She wanted me to get under the rug with her but the thunder could go on for ages. Apart from feeling ridiculous, I didn't really want to spend the entire evening sitting in the car park under a travel rug so I decided to come in and do the shopping on my own.'

'Is your car the blue Ford Cortina?'

'Yes it is. How did you know?'

'I saw a strange shape moving about on the back seat as I walked past. At first, I thought it was a dog that had got tangled up in a travel rug but then a woman's head popped out. It gave me quite a shock.'

'That would have been my mother,' said Harriet, raising her eyes in mild embarrassment and chuckling at the same time.

I was concerned to hear that her mother was so afraid of thunder. 'Will she be all right? It must be awful for her if she's really scared. Perhaps you ought to get back to her right away.'

Harriet brushed off the suggestion. 'She'll be fine, though I don't suppose she'll be happy about driving home unless the thunder stops.'

'So what will you do? As you said, the thunder could go on for some time.'

'I'll have to drive, though she's probably as scared of my driving as she is of thunder.'

'Why, aren't you very good?'

'Shall we say, Mr Derwent, I'm a bit lacking in experience.'

'Please call me Justin. Mr Derwent sounds so formal.'

'But you're my dentist. Come to think of it, you smell like a dentist. Oh, I'm sorry, Mr Derwent, I mean, Justin, I shouldn't have said that – it was very rude of me.'

It was my turn to laugh. 'It's the oil of cloves – the characteristic smell of a dental surgery – it gets into everything and I'm not your dentist any more so it's all right for you to call me Justin.'

'All right then: Justin. I didn't mean to insult you – really I didn't – it's a nice smell.'

'You were telling me about your driving.'

Harriet looked more serious. 'Yes. I only passed my test a few months ago. My mother was praying that I wouldn't because she didn't think I'd had enough lessons. To be honest, I don't think I was really ready and I didn't expect to pass but miraculously I did.'

'Perhaps you charmed the examiner.'

'I don't know about that but my mother was very upset that I passed. She thought it would be a good idea if I carried on having lessons.'

'So did you?'

'No. Being a student I couldn't really afford it. I didn't see much point in having more lessons because I felt sure I knew what I should be doing – it's just that I wasn't very good at putting it into practice. I decided that all I needed was a bit more experience. Anyway, one evening I borrowed her car to take a friend out and I realised that I needed petrol. When I found a petrol station I drove in at about thirty miles an hour and without slowing down, I crashed straight into the pumps. I don't know what came over me but I made

120

a real mess of my mother's car – and the pumps. My friend went very pale and my little dog dived under the seat, shaking.'

'Oh dear. Not a very good start to your driving career but we all do silly things when we've just passed the driving test and we go out on our own for the first time.'

'Maybe, but that was particularly stupid and of course it played right into my mother's hands, who was then even more convinced I should have more lessons. The garage owner wasn't very pleased with me either. He shot out of his office and sprayed everything with foam from a fire extinguisher, then he started shouting at me. He said he knew it would be a woman driver and that only a woman could be so incompetent as to drive in there at that speed and not slow down. He said I could have killed someone and I obviously wasn't fit to be on the road. He was in an awful temper and his face was so red I thought he was going to burst a blood vessel.'

'What did you say?'

'I didn't say anything. I did the only thing a woman can do in situations like that – I burst into tears.'

'I can see that you're making good use of your knowledge of psychology. Did crying help to calm him down?'

'Yes. He then started to feel sorry for me, though my mother was somewhat less forgiving. Anyway, the car and the petrol pumps have now been straightened out and I learnt a very important lesson.'

'That it's best to slow down when driving into a petrol station?'

'No. That bursting into tears can get you out of all sorts of trouble.'

Harriet's eyes twinkled again and I found myself completely captivated by her. There was another loud clap of thunder and my thoughts turned once again to her mother.

'Your mother won't like that. Shouldn't you be getting back to her?'

Harriet didn't seem in any particular hurry to end our conversation. 'She'll be all right. I'll go to her in a minute. Tell me, Mr Derwent, I mean Justin, what made you want to be a dentist?'

'I suppose I wanted to do something practical. I tried working in an office and I hated it so I had to find something that would combine study and academic achievement with working with my hands, and there aren't very many jobs that allow you to do that.'

'I think dentistry is a very glamorous profession.'

'Do you really? It's not very glamorous when you're up to your elbows in blood trying to remove a wisdom tooth that refuses to budge.'

'It isn't often like that, is it? I think it's extremely skilful to be able to carry out such intricate work in the confines of someone's mouth. You are helping people, improving their appearance and curing pain and suffering. It must be very rewarding.'

'It can be, but it can also be very demanding. As a student of psychology you must know that dealing with people can be difficult at times and when they're nervous, as they usually are at the dentist's, their behaviour can sometimes be out of character. Anyway, what are you hoping to do when you leave university?'

'I'm not entirely sure but I shall probably go into teaching. I'm taking a teaching certificate in addition to my degree, in case that's the way I decide to go.'

'Can't psychologists earn huge amounts of money providing psychotherapy?'

Harriet didn't seem to be particularly excited at the prospect. 'Yes they can, especially in America but I've no desire to leave England and money isn't everything. To be honest, I really like it here. I don't like Southampton very much – it's too big and busy. I'm much happier in the country and I think this area has everything: it's not too built up; there's lots of lovely open countryside and it's not too far from the coast.'

'So you'll be looking for a job in this area, will you?'

'Yes. I don't know if I'll be able to find one but I shall certainly try.'

'Well I wish you luck. I hope you find something suitable.'

'And perhaps you can become my regular dentist?'

'I would be very happy to have you as a patient.'

There was another intense flash of lightning followed immediately by a peal of thunder which seemed to shake the very foundations of the building in which we were standing.

'I suppose I'd better get back to my mother,' said Harriet. 'It's been lovely talking to you, Justin. I wish we could talk longer.'

'I've enjoyed talking to you too, Harriet. I hope your mother is all right.'

'She'll be okay. I hope to see you again sometime, Justin. Goodbye.'

122

'Goodbye, Harriet. Oh I nearly forgot to ask – how are the mouth ulcers?'

'Much less painful. They obviously haven't gone completely yet but the mouthwash you prescribed for me seems to be working. Thank you so much for seeing me.'

'It was my pleasure. Take care and good luck with your exams.'

She left the shop and just before she disappeared from view she looked back and waved to me. I immediately cursed myself for not asking her out. She said she would have liked to have talked for longer so surely she would have agreed to go out for a drink with me. There was something about her that I found most appealing. I had never experienced quite the same feeling about anyone else before, so why on earth did I let the chance to get to know her better slip away from me. Richard Darcy said that if you liked the look of someone you couldn't afford to miss the opportunity, and his words were ringing in my ears. I certainly liked the look of Harriet Brooks and whilst I had my reasons for not asking her out when she came to see me as a patient, there was no excuse for messing up a second golden opportunity. I thought that the chances of seeing her at some time in the future were probably very slim. I couldn't believe how utterly foolish I'd been and I would probably go on regretting it for a long time to come.

CHAPTER NINETEEN

I was astounded at the speed with which Wendy settled in as my new nurse. I thought it would take at least a few weeks before she became familiar with my way of working and to learn where every piece of equipment and all the materials I used were kept but she accomplished it in a couple of days. She seemed to anticipate my every move and I found that she was constantly one step ahead so that when I needed her to pass me something she already had it to hand without my having to ask for it. When Ingrid first came to work for me she had no previous dental nursing experience and had gradually become very proficient and I was sorry to see her go. Wendy however, was super-efficient from the start because of her previous experience. Not only was she a good nurse but she was also liked by the patients because she was so friendly and cheerful, and she was a pleasure to work with. I told Spencer how pleased I was with her and not unexpectedly, he tried to take credit for having chosen so wisely. However, he knew that I was aware of the circumstances by which he found her and that, in truth, he had had very little to do with it so he wasn't able to gloat too much.

I looked at my list of appointments for the morning and was surprised to see that the first patient was Mr H. Rutherford.

'Not young Harold?' Wendy queried.

'It must be, though according to Spencer there's very little chance that he'll turn up but I hope he does because he's booked in for three quarters of an hour, though I don't know why he's been given an appointment of that length just for a check-up.'

Beryl suddenly appeared and provided the answer. 'His father phoned up yesterday and asked if you could see him urgently because he needs some fillings in his front teeth and he wants them done as soon as possible. Mrs Soper had just cancelled her nine o'clock appointment because she's ill and as you had three quarters of an hour clear, I gave it to him.'

'He's not due for another ten minutes so we can't assume he's failed his appointment yet,' Wendy pointed out.

Beryl continued. 'I'm really here to tell you that Reverend Jenkinson has just turned up and wonders if you could see him for a few minutes.'

'Oh dear, I hope he hasn't got pain again,' I replied. 'You'd better go and fetch him Wendy.'

'I'm awfully sorry to trouble you again, Justin,' sighed Reverend Jenkinson.

'Has it started hurting again,' I asked with some concern.

'Oh no; there's no pain. Mr Padginton's brown paste cured it completely. No, I'm here because my lower denture is now very loose. It's floating about and makes talking difficult. I wouldn't worry about it but I'm officiating at a funeral tomorrow and it might destroy the solemnity of the occasion if my lower denture jumps out in the middle of the service. Is there anything you can do to stick it down?'

'Ah yes, I see the problem. What we need to do is to add another tooth on to your denture so that it fits tightly against the tooth behind. I'll need to take an impression for the technician to work with and you'll need to leave your denture with me. If you'd like to take a seat I'll take the impression now.'

'Surely you can't get it done before tomorrow, can you?'

'Yes I can. I'll phone the technician and get him to pick it up this morning and he'll bring it back this afternoon so you can collect it about five o'clock. Will that be all right?'

'That's marvellous, Justin. I'm so grateful to you. I have to say you offer a wonderful service here.'

'I'm very pleased to be able to help. I hope the funeral is less eventful than the wedding you conducted recently.'

'My goodness, so do I. That was awful. I wouldn't be surprised if they're in the process of getting a divorce now. You don't expect the tribulations of married life to begin at the church ceremony, do you? Are you married, Justin?'

'No I'm not married.'

'Are you not? Is there someone special in your life?'

'Not really.'

'Well I don't know how old you are exactly but you have obviously completed a lengthy university course and you are now settled into your career so I think the time has come for you to be looking for a lifelong companion.'

'Do you think so?'

'I most certainly do.'

'It has to be the right person though.'

'Oh indeed it does but I can thoroughly recommend it. I've been very fortunate twice in my life. My first wife sadly died and it took me a long time to get over it but then I met Edna, my present wife, who turned out to be just as wonderful. Life is so much more enjoyable when you have someone to share it with.'

'I'll remember what you've said, Reverend Jenkinson.'

'You do that, Justin and please call me Walter.'

I quickly took an impression of Reverend Jenkinson's lower jaw and Wendy escorted him to the front door where she met Mr Rutherford and another gentleman, who she assumed was 'young Harold'. Spencer had told us that 'young Harold' wasn't exactly in the first bloom of youth but we still had quite a shock when we saw him, as his demeanour was that of someone much older than his years. His back was stooped and he shuffled along as if propelled by Mr Rutherford. He appeared to be very unsteady on his feet and progress up the stairs was very slow and laboured. Mr Rutherford held tightly on to his arm to prevent him from falling down.

When he was safely installed in my dental chair and I got nearer to him the smell of alcohol pervaded my nostrils and I began to understand why he was looking so debilitated and unsteady.

'You'll need to treat him very gently, Mr Derwent,' Mr Rutherford advised. 'He finds situations like this very difficult. Not so long ago I discovered that he was taking to the brandy bottle if he had to face something which made him nervous. I can tell you I soon put a stop to that – I'm not having a son of mine drinking! I've stopped him smoking as well; I think it's a disgusting habit, not only is it very unhealthy but it's also a terrible waste of money.'

I looked at the fingers on Harold's right hand and saw that they were stained brown. It seemed that Mr Rutherford had been less successful than he thought in curbing Harold's smoking and drinking.

'He wants his front teeth filled, Mr Derwent. They don't look very good at the moment with big black holes in them and I think it's affecting his confidence. He seems to be very self-conscious and avoids meeting people. If anyone speaks to him he puts his hand over his mouth before he answers them. He's always been a bit on the shy side but I think his teeth are affecting his life very badly now. I want you to do something with them.'

Harold hadn't said a word so far and every time I tried to speak to him his father answered for him. I decided that I would have to separate them if I wanted to establish a relationship with the patient. 'Would you mind taking a seat in the waiting room whilst I treat Harold, please Mr Rutherford?' I requested.

'I think I ought to stay here with him. He might need me.'

I could see that Mr Rutherford was not going to be moved easily and Wendy came to the rescue. 'Mr Derwent prefers to be alone when he's treating his patients, Mr Rutherford, why don't you come with me and I'll make you a cup of tea. I think they'll get on much better if we leave them to it.' She spoke softly and caringly but her manner was firm and when she smiled at him he seemed to find it difficult to resist. He turned and left the surgery without another word.

Harold changed completely as soon as his father had left. He livened up and became quite coherent once I started talking to him on a one to one basis. There was no doubt that he'd been drinking but it didn't appear to have adversely affected his ability to hold a rational conversation.

'I'd like you to improve the appearance of my front teeth,' he explained. 'They look awful with these holes in them. Can you fill them?'

I examined them carefully and it was quite clear that the cavities were not new; they must have been present for many years as they were very stained.

'They are long-standing cavities, Mr Rutherford and there's a lot of tooth tissue missing. It's a pity you didn't come sooner to get them filled.'

'It wasn't important until now.'

'So what's changed?'

Harold looked slightly uncomfortable and paused for some moments before replying. 'If I tell you something will you promise not to say anything to my father?'

'Of course; anything you say to me is entirely confidential.'

'You do promise?'

'Yes I promise.'

'I've got a girlfriend – well she isn't exactly a girl she's in her fifties but you know what I mean.'

'Oh I see, and your father doesn't know about her?'

'That's right and I don't want him to – he wouldn't approve. He knows I'm self-conscious about my teeth but he doesn't know the real reason.'

I was going to tell him that as he was sixty-two years of age, surely he was old enough to make his own decisions in life but then I decided it was none of my business.

'All right, Mr Rutherford, I'll see what I can do with your front teeth. I can certainly improve their appearance but because the cavities are so large the fillings might not stay in very well.'

'I understand, Mr Derwent, but I would be grateful if you could do something to make them look better.'

Thirty five minutes later the appearance of Harold's front teeth had been transformed. He proved to be a co-operative patient and I had no difficulty in treating him. I polished off all the tobacco staining, excavated the discoloured and carious dentine and filled the cavities with tooth-coloured filling material. Harold was surprised and extremely pleased when I held the mirror for him to inspect the results.

Wendy allowed Mr Rutherford senior to return to the surgery to be reunited with Harold.

'Let me have a look at them, son. That's better! My goodness, don't they look good? Have you thanked Mr Derwent for making you handsome again?' he effused.

Harold immediately shut down again understandably embarrassed that his father was treating him like a five-year-old. He reverted to being a downtrodden, silent introvert and I felt so sorry for him because I was sure there was an intelligent person inside him trying to get out but unable to do so because of his overbearing father.

I thought about him a lot during the rest of the day. It seemed unbelievable that he had been dominated by his father all his life and had never felt able to break away. The situation was so far advanced now it seemed unlikely that Harold would ever summon up the courage to say how he really felt and to admit that he was still smoking and drinking in spite of being forbidden to do so and to come out into the open with the fact that he now had a lady friend.

I was still thinking about him at five o'clock, just after I'd finished treating my last patient of the day, when Wendy came into my surgery to tell me that Mr Rutherford was on the phone and wanted to speak to me.

'Senior or junior?' I asked.

'Senior of course,' she replied with a grin.

'Of course, how silly of me to ask.'

'Hello, Mr Rutherford, what can I do for you?'

'It's about Harold's teeth.'

'What about them? Isn't he pleased with his fillings?'

'He thinks they look all right but he's just discovered that he can't whistle the dog now the gaps have been filled. I don't know what you can do about it but it's a serious disadvantage.'

I really didn't know quite what to say. It just made me realise that however hard you try to do your best to please, there is always going to be some unforeseen reason why someone will see it as not being good enough. I'd had a busy day and I was tired. It was upsetting and slightly annoying to think that I had given him an appointment at short notice and tried very hard to help him when he asked me to but it seemed my efforts were not really appreciated.

My reply was polite but fairly blunt. 'I can drill the fillings out again if you want me to but you asked me to improve his appearance and that's what I've done. You and Harold have to decide what's more important – his appearance or his ability to whistle the dog.'

CHAPTER TWENTY

I thought about Harriet a lot during the week and she was still on my mind when I went to meet Sarah on the Saturday evening. I kept telling myself that it was most unlikely that I would meet her again so why was I wasting my time dwelling on what might have been? In reality, I knew hardly anything about her, or she about me, and there was absolutely no guarantee we would be any good together in the long term or that she would even want to strike up any sort of relationship other than dentist/patient. She probably had a boyfriend anyway.

Nevertheless, I had to admit that if I had been given a choice, I would have chosen to go out with Harriet rather than Sarah and I wondered if, out of fairness, I ought to tell Sarah how I felt. I decided, however, that there wasn't any point because there wasn't really anything to tell. I had had a professional encounter and a subsequent casual meeting with a girl to whom I had taken a liking but probably everyone, even married people, occasionally meet members of the opposite sex to whom they are attracted but if nothing more comes of it, then it's hardly newsworthy. Secondly, if I did tell Sarah, then it would certainly ruin our evening out together and there didn't seem much point in doing that. I decided that I wouldn't say anything and I would do my best to put Harriet out of my mind. The only niggling thought that remained was that, in view of the fact Harriet drew my attention so quickly and easily, perhaps it indicated there was something lacking in my feelings for Sarah.

I decided I was becoming far too philosophical about the whole thing. I liked Sarah and as I rang her doorbell I resolved to do my very best to make the evening as enjoyable as possible.

She greeted me warmly with a kiss. 'It's lovely to see you again, Justin. How are you?'

'I'm fine thank you, Sarah. How are you?'

'Better for seeing you. It seems ages since I last saw you.'

Sarah's dogs left me in no doubt that they were pleased to see me too. They came to me wagging their tails furiously and licking my hands with great enthusiasm. It was a wonderful welcome and made me feel very special.

'It's quite a pleasant evening now, unlike last Sunday. I don't know about you but I feel in need of some fresh air. How do you feel about a long walk before we find a nice little pub somewhere for a drink and a bite to eat?'

'That would be really nice,' replied Sarah. 'I also feel in need of fresh air. I do have a small favour to ask, though. It's the birthday of one of my mother's friends on Tuesday and she asked if I could go to the newsagents down the road to buy a birthday card. Would you mind awfully if we called in there on our way out?'

'Of course not. What time do they close?'

'They're open until about nine o'clock. I'm sorry to ask you, Justin, but my mother hasn't been too well and she hasn't had a chance to get a card.'

'That's all right, it's no problem.'

'Thank you so much.'

It was quite busy at the newsagent's. They obviously had a flourishing evening trade, being the only shop that stayed open until late. At first I thought I wouldn't be able to park anywhere near the shop but people were coming and going quite quickly and someone drove off just as we arrived, which enabled me to nip into a space almost directly outside.

'I won't be a minute,' said Sarah.

I got out of the car and stepped onto the pavement. There was a refreshing breeze which gently ruffled my hair and the evening sun felt warm on my face. It was such an agreeable change from the stormy conditions we had experienced for the past two weeks and I leaned back against the nearside front wing enjoying the moment. I closed my eyes and my mind began to drift.

I'm not sure how long I stayed there; it couldn't have been more than a few minutes before I was awakened from my trance when I felt Sarah's lips on mine.

'I'm sorry,' she said 'but I couldn't resist doing that.'

'Don't apologise,' I replied, surprised by her sudden, spontaneous display of affection. 'It was a very pleasant way to be brought back from my daydream.'

Before she could say any more, her attention was snatched away by something she witnessed happening behind me on the other side of the road.

'My God, that car just mounted the pavement and narrowly missed the streetlamp,' she exclaimed. 'The driver must be drunk or something.'

I turned round to see a blue Ford Cortina driven by a young woman speed away down the road. I didn't get a good look at the driver but it was definitely a young woman and I suddenly remembered that Harriet's mother owned a blue Ford Cortina. In fact I saw it parked outside the supermarket when I met Harriet earlier in the week. I was fairly sure it was the same car. Could it possibly have been Harriet driving? If it was, then it was an amazing coincidence that she should happen to be driving past at that very moment. And why was she driving so badly? She had said that her driving wasn't very good but there must have been a reason for her mounting the pavement. Something must have distracted her. Could it possibly have been that she recognised me and that's what distracted her? My heart sank as I realised that if she had recognised me, then she would have seen Sarah kissing me. Could that be what caused her to mount the pavement? The worst part about it was that she would now have reached the conclusion that I had a girlfriend, so even if she had been at all interested in me she would surely decide there was no point in taking it any further. Any chance I might have had of getting to know her better would now be completely ruined. I couldn't believe I could be that unlucky.

Sarah sensed that I was deep in thought about the incident.

'Do you know the driver?' she demanded.

'I didn't really see her.'

'Do you know anyone who owns a blue Ford Cortina?'

I hesitated. 'No, I don't think so,' I replied unconvincingly. I tried to ease my feeling of guilt by telling myself that I wasn't really lying because it was Harriet's mother who owned the car and as I hadn't actually met her, it was true to say I didn't know her.

'You don't sound very sure.'

132

'I am sure. In any case if it was someone I know, or someone who knows me, they would have stopped or waved or blown their horn, wouldn't they?'

'I don't know. They might not if they hadn't expected to see you with me.'

'What do you mean, Sarah?'

'Nothing. I'm just a bit mystified as to why she was driving so erratically. Something distracted her, that's for sure and I'd love to know what it was.'

'I think you're reading too much into it. She's probably just a typical woman driver who had her mind on other things and wasn't concentrating on her driving.'

CHAPTER TWENTY ONE

'Good morning, Justin,' Spencer shouted as soon I stepped inside the front entrance hall.

The excitement in his voice was unmistakeable and he was calling from inside the old waiting room; the room which was to become his new surgery. I gathered from this that he had begun to get the room ready for the change and I was anxious to find out what he had done. Perhaps he was planning the layout of his new surgery and trying to visualise how it would look with some new equipment set up in there. The first thing I noticed was that there was a new door on the room, which surprised me. To my mind, it wasn't an improvement because the old door had panels and was rather attractive whilst the new replacement was completely plain, uninteresting plywood with a small wired glass window, the reason for which was a mystery to me.

'A new door I see, Spencer.'

'Yes it's all to do with fire regulations. This is a fire check door and has a half-hour rating.'

'Who said you needed to fit a fire door?'

'Well no-one actually but I thought it would be a good idea.'

'And what's the purpose of the window?'

'I assume it's so that you can see a fire in the room from outside or if anyone is trapped inside.'

'The old door was more attractive. Did you buy this one?'

'No I had it in my workshop. I can't remember where it came from originally; I've had it a long time.'

'What did you do with the old one?'

'My friend Geoff bought it.'

The situation was becoming clear to me. 'I get it,' I conjectured. 'Geoff took a fancy to the old door and made you an offer you couldn't refuse. You let him have it because you knew you had another door you could replace it with; is that it?'

'More or less,' Spencer replied quietly. 'Anyway, go in and see what I've done.'

I went in, expecting to see a bare room with perhaps some electric cables and water pipes which had been installed to provide services to a new chair and dental unit. I knew that Spencer had intended to spend the weekend working on it but I felt sure that the whole job would probably take quite a long time and as far as I was aware Spencer hadn't yet decided on what equipment to buy. It came, therefore, as a great surprise to me when I saw before me the entire contents of his old surgery laid out exactly as they had been in his room upstairs. The same antiquated, upright leather dental chair and the same old drill unit and operating light all set up in exactly the same relative positions. The view out of the window was obviously different being at ground level, so this and the more elaborate fireplace were the only things to indicate that it wasn't the same room that he had worked in previously. Not a single item had been upgraded or renewed. I couldn't believe it.

'I'm up and running,' he declared with great enthusiasm.

'I thought you were going to buy some new equipment,' I gasped, incredulous that he could even consider retaining all his old equipment. I thought that moving his surgery would have given him a golden opportunity to bring things up to date.

'Yes, I thought about it and I did look at some but I just didn't like what I saw. It's all so badly made – it won't last five minutes. In the end I decided I was better off keeping what I already had.'

I was still aghast at the speed at which Spencer had been able to move his entire surgery. 'How did you manage to move everything down here so quickly? Did you get help from the dental supply company's engineer?'

'No, I got some of my friends from the Sports Car Club to come and help me. The dental company's engineer wanted a ridiculous hourly rate, which would have been even higher if he'd worked over the weekend. I certainly wasn't prepared to pay that.'

'I'm amazed that you managed to move everything so quickly and get it all set up with the plumbing and electrics. But I did think that moving the surgery would have been an ideal opportunity to upgrade your equipment.'

'It doesn't need upgrading, Justin. It works perfectly well and will continue to do so for many years to come. I did get one thing new, though. What do you think to this?'

He opened one of his low-level cupboard doors to reveal an old electric motor which sat alongside a large metal canister. There were numerous wires and tubes coiled up and lying on top.

'What is it?' I asked.

'It's a high-speed aspirator. I decided my old saliva ejector was a bit feeble and I needed something that would suck out water much more quickly. It's so important to keep the operating field clear of blood, saliva, water from the drill and also debris, so you can see exactly what you're doing. That's what this will do.'

My attention was drawn to the scratched paint on the canister and the accumulated dust on the electric motor. 'It doesn't look very new,' I remarked.

'Well it isn't brand new. I bought it from a dentist in Devon. It was advertised for sale in one of the dental magazines. He assured me it's in perfect working order and I've no reason to think otherwise. I haven't had time to set it up yet but it won't take long – it will soon be in operation.'

'The canister doesn't look very big. It will soon fill up and you'll have to stop work to empty it, which will be a very messy job. Don't you think it will be rather inconvenient?'

'No, no, Justin. You don't have to empty it very often. It's just a separation canister – it separates the liquids from the solids so waste amalgam collects inside it and has to be emptied perhaps once a month. The liquid drains out of the bottom.'

'And where does it go?'

'Into the drains. It's brilliant because I can sell the waste amalgam, which will collect in the canister, as scrap, whereas, at the moment, it all gets washed away down the drain. Think of all the precious silver that's being washed away and lost forever. The money I'll get from selling the waste will pay for this piece of equipment in no time.'

'You don't get much for waste amalgam.'

'I know you don't,' Spencer agreed, 'but I didn't pay much for this either. I think it was an absolute bargain and will prove to be an extremely useful addition to my surgery equipment. I'm always looking for ways of moving the practice forward and I think this will do just that.'

I nearly choked at Spencer's claim and still found it hard to believe that he had moved all his equipment lock, stock and barrel downstairs and had refused to replace any of it even though it was antiquated.

'I've also, with the help of my friends from the Sports Car Club, redecorated the cloakroom. Come and look at it.'

'It was in need of brightening up – I always thought the walls were too dark for a small room. What colour did you paint it?'

'I didn't use paint,' he replied haughtily, 'I had a brilliant idea which I think is quite innovative. As you know I subscribe to the National Geographic magazine and have done for years. It's a first class magazine though I rarely get time to read it, unfortunately. Anyway, with each issue they have been giving away maps of different countries of the world. It's a great shame that no-one really studies these maps and I decided it would be a great idea to decorate the cloakroom with them so you can sit on the toilet and plan a journey round the world.'

'Not to mention the fact that it saved you from buying paint or wallpaper?'

'Well I suppose that was a consideration but what do you think of it?' he enquired as he opened the door and stepped aside to let me experience the full impact of his handiwork.

'It's certainly different,' I exclaimed. I suppose I had imagined that the maps would be quite small and framed with maybe two or three on each side of the room and surrounded by an area where the painted wall formed a background but it wasn't like that at all. The maps were pasted directly on to the walls and butted together so there was no exposed blank wall whatsoever from floor to ceiling over the entire room. Once I got over the initial shock my next observation was that there had been little attention paid to global layout. Some of the maps had had to be cut in order to cover the entire wall space and consequently, in one corner, part of New Zealand overlapped Africa and in another, the North Pole was only a few degrees of latitude north of the equator.

'It gives a new meaning to the concept of continental drift,' I remarked.

'Ah, well yes,' Spencer agreed. 'I had to take a few liberties in order to cover the walls fully but don't you think the overall effect is impressive?'

'Oh very,' I answered with sincerity. 'So when do you think I will be moving downstairs?'

'Soon, Justin, because I want to keep the whole practice together. I don't think it's good for part of it to be upstairs and part downstairs. I would, however, like a bit of breathing space before undertaking the next phase of the move because it's been very tiring for me to get this far in such a short time. I've been working late into the night for the past two weeks and I'm feeling quite exhausted.'

'I know you've worked hard, Spencer, to achieve so much in such a short time but it would be better if my surgery were downstairs now.'

'Exactly, Justin, and I promise I'll start moving everything out of the sitting room as soon as I've got my breath back.'

'I've been thinking,' I began, wondering if now was a good time to say what I had in mind. 'I've been wondering how you would feel about it if I were to buy some new equipment for my new surgery. I know you're happy to work with old equipment but we had the very latest at the dental hospital. I trained on it and in spite of what you think, I believe it has many advantages and I'm sure it would enable me to work much more efficiently.'

'You want to buy it?'

'Yes. I'm quite happy here and I can't see me moving. I know it's unusual for an associate to buy his own equipment but I'm willing to do so if you will let me. If, for any reason, I do leave, we can come to some arrangement about what to do with the equipment. You could buy it from me if you wish, or I could take it with me and if you hang on to the equipment I'm using at present, you could always reinstall that.'

Spencer looked thoughtful for a few moments. 'I really can't understand why you want to waste your money on new equipment. There's nothing wrong with the equipment you're using at present, is there?'

'There's nothing really wrong with it, it's just that it's not like the equipment I trained on and it isn't ideally suited to working with the patient lying flat.'

'Patients don't like lying flat, in fact, they hate it. At least that's the feeling I get from talking to them about it.'

'I know older people generally don't like to lie too far back but that's because they haven't been used to it. When someone starts to tell me they don't want to lie flat, I say to them "when I go to the

138

dentist, I'm more concerned about his comfort than my own so I prefer to let him decide what position he wants me in – I'm sure I get a better job done that way. And if you go into hospital for an operation you don't start telling the surgeon you're not happy to lie flat, so why tell the dentist?" Young people don't seem to mind and whilst the average age of my patients might be about seventy-five at present, I hope it won't always be like that. You say you want the practice to move forward and as I see it, that means getting rid of equipment that looks as if it has just come out of a museum. I'm hoping to increase the amount of crown and bridgework I do, which can be very lucrative, but it's very tiring and difficult to do good work if you are straining your back to see into the patient's mouth.'

'It's just that I think modern equipment is a load of rubbish but if that's really what you want to spend your money on, I don't have any objections. It is, however, very good to know that you are happy here, Justin.'

He paused again briefly.

'It's quite gratifying to hear that you're prepared to make what would be quite a big commitment and I see it as a vote of confidence in this practice. When my father retired and I knew that I would have to employ an associate I was worried it might be difficult to find someone who would be prepared to work here for any length of time. I think it's very bad for a dental practice if dentists are constantly leaving and patients have to see someone new every time they come for treatment. Stability is most important. I feel that you have fitted into the practice very well – patients like you and you are attracting new ones in your own right. I have been very thankful for this but, at the back of my mind, I had the niggling worry that you might want to move on, perhaps to a more glamorous practice.'

'I've no plans to move on, Spencer. I like working here. I think you and I get on well together and you more or less let me do whatever I want. I like the area and I've made a few friends. I've no great ambitions and having sampled a taste of country life I certainly wouldn't want to move back to a city.'

'It's good to hear that, Justin, and I'm so pleased you feel settled here. Perhaps this means that the time has come for me to review our professional relationship and consider an expense sharing agreement of some sort or even a partnership instead of an associateship. I'll think about it. As far as your new equipment is concerned, as I said, I've no objections to your getting some but I would strongly advise you to be careful because in my opinion not only is it rubbish, but it's very expensive rubbish.'

'That's great, Spencer. Thank you very much, I'll do some research before I make any decisions and I am very interested and delighted at the idea of an improvement to my status in the practice.'

Our conversation ended there because Wendy came in to tell me that my first patient had arrived.

'It's Mr Lannigan,' she announced, 'he's a new patient, you haven't seen him before. He's been recommended to come and see you by one of his friends. I wouldn't upset him if I were you; he's about six foot four tall and must weigh at least twenty stone. He seems friendly enough though, he's probably what you would call a gentle giant.'

He was already sitting in my chair when I got to the surgery so I wasn't able to appreciate his enormous stature but I could see that his huge body filled my chair completely.

'Good morning, Mr Lannigan. What can I do for you?'

'I want you take out all my teeth, Mr Derwent, please.'

'All of them? Why what's wrong with them?'

'There's nothing wrong with them at the moment but I'm sure it's only a matter of time before they start to give trouble.'

'Not necessarily. Have you had trouble with them in the past?'

'No not really but as I said, they're bound to give trouble sooner or later and by having them out now I can avoid that happening.'

'Can I have a look?'

He obligingly opened his cavernous mouth to reveal a full set of very strong and healthy-looking teeth set in equally healthy-looking gums.

'You've got excellent teeth, Mr Lannigan, it would be quite wrong to extract them.'

'I've made my mind up, Mr Derwent. I want to get rid of them. My father had terrible trouble with his teeth when he got to fifty and I don't want to suffer in the same way. I'll avoid that if I have them out now.'

'I'm sorry, Mr Lannigan, but I can't agree with you. You have very good teeth and you appear to look after them well so there's no reason at all why they should give you trouble later on. If you get them checked regularly by a dentist, there's every chance they'll serve you well for the rest of your life.'

'But you can't be sure of that can you, Mr Derwent?'

'Fairly sure.'

'That's not really good enough. No, I've thought it through very carefully and I've decided the only way I can be sure I won't get trouble later on is to have all my teeth out now.'

I was finding it difficult to understand why a young man with healthy teeth would be so intent on having them all extracted and I continued to try to dissuade him.

'Many people who are having trouble with their teeth think that all their problems will be over if they have their teeth out. It simply isn't true. What they don't realise is that they will just be replacing one set of problems with much worse ones. In your case it makes even less sense because you aren't actually having trouble. The best false teeth in the world are nowhere near as good as your own. Have you thought what it will be like to have false teeth?'

'I'll get used to them. My father did.'

'You might get used to them but it takes time, and there are some people who never really adjust to them. They are nowhere near as efficient as your own teeth, you know. You are a big, strong man with powerful jaws and it's quite possible that you would be constantly breaking your dentures.'

'You won't change my mind, Mr Derwent. Will you do as I ask and take them all out for me?'

'I'm sorry, Mr Lannigan but it would be against my professional judgement. I don't think it would be in your best interests so I'm not prepared to do it for you.'

'They're my teeth. Surely I can do what I like with them.'

'That's true and you might find a dentist who is prepared to do it but I think it would be wrong and I feel sure that one day you would regret it.'

'So you are refusing to help me?'

'I don't think I would be helping you if I took out all your teeth.'

Mr Lannigan stared vacantly at me for a few moments and I could see that his eyes were beginning to fill with tears.

'Please do as I ask, Mr Derwent. I've thought about it very carefully and I'm sure that having my teeth out would be the right thing for me.'

I could see that I was getting nowhere with him and time was running on. I was quite sure I would be doing him a great disservice if I were to take out all his teeth but quite clearly he did not see it that way and was equally sure that having them extracted was the right course of action.

'What I suggest, Mr Lannigan, is that you make another appointment to come and see me and I'll carry out a full examination of your teeth and take some X-rays so that I can assess the likelihood of you getting problems with them in the future. In the meantime I want you to think very carefully about what I've told you. I want you to consider what it would be like to go around for six months with no teeth at all whilst we wait for your gums to heal because we wouldn't be able to fit you with false teeth immediately. It would then take several months before you got used to them and remember that you'll never be able to eat as well with them as you can with your own teeth.'

His face brightened a little. 'So you're not saying definitely you won't do it, Mr Derwent?'

'I'm not making any promises. I just want you to go away and think a bit more about it. Make an appointment for two weeks' time and we'll discuss it further then.'

He stood up and towered above me like a giant oak tree. His shoulders looked as if they were strong enough to hold up a ten ton lorry, and he held out his huge hand which totally engulfed mine in a ferociously firm handshake.

As soon as he had gone, Wendy turned to me with an expression of incredulity and dismay. 'You aren't going to change your mind about taking out his teeth, are you, Justin?'

'Of course not. I'm sure it would be completely the wrong thing to do. The question is how can I convince him that it's not a good idea? The other point which I haven't mentioned yet is that he is so big and strong, and he's a young man. I'll bet his teeth are set in concrete and it would be a devil of a job to get out his upper canines and his molars. Any dentist who tries to take them all out in one go is going to be in for a very tough time – I certainly wouldn't want to attempt it.'

Most patients are very anxious to keep their teeth and I found it difficult to understand why Mr Lannigan felt the way he did. It seemed, however, that he had made up his mind and it wasn't going to be easy to change his views. I thought about it a lot during the rest of the morning and wondered how I was going to handle his next appointment. What could I say or do to convince him that he really ought to be thankful he had good teeth and that he should definitely not get rid of them.

I was still thinking about it when Wendy came into the surgery looking extremely pale and shaken.

'What's the matter, Wendy, you look as if you've just seen a ghost?'

'Something terrible has happened,' she said. 'It's Mr Lannigan. He's dead.'

'Dead? That's not possible; he only left here less than two hours ago. How do you know about it? Was he involved in an accident?'

'Beryl has just taken a phone call from the coroner's office. They wanted to know who had an appointment for eleven o'clock on the 28th of this month. Apparently he just collapsed and died in the centre of Crewkerne and he wasn't carrying any means of identification. The only thing he had on him was his appointment card so they phoned here to find out who he was. Spencer has someone booked in at that time on that day but his patient is an old lady. They also said it was a great big man, so it must be Mr Lannigan.'

'That's unbelievable – he looked so strong and healthy.'

'I know,' sighed Wendy. 'It's very hard to believe. It just goes to show that none of us knows what's in store for us. If it can happen to someone as young and strong as Mr Lannigan, it could happen to anyone.'

'He obviously wasn't as strong and healthy as he looked. I'm just glad I didn't carry out any treatment on him or give him an injection because I would worry that I might have been responsible in some way.'

'Gosh, Justin, I hadn't thought of that. That would have been terrible.'

CHAPTER TWENTY TWO

I found it very hard to forget about Mr Lannigan. It just didn't seem possible that he could leave my surgery, apparently fit and well, drive to Crewkerne, and then drop dead. He seemed perfectly all right when he left. If he had been old and infirm it would have been easier to accept and I found myself thinking there must be some sort of mistake and that he would probably turn up for his appointment on the 28th. I wondered if Wendy felt the same because I noticed she didn't take his name out of the appointment book. In reality, however, the facts were clear, and sad though it was, I had to believe it had actually happened.

I tried to put it out of my mind and suddenly my attention was seized by Mrs Crossley's indignant outburst. 'I don't believe it!' she screamed. 'That just about takes the biscuit. If you ask me he's got a bloomin' nerve.' She was in the process of cleaning the floor of Spencer's surgery and just happened to look out of the window to see a man, presumably a patient, get out of his car and walk to the door of the practice.

'What on earth's the matter Mrs Crossley,' I enquired, wondering what could possibly have upset the normally placid housekeeper to erupt in this way.

'It's my doctor, Dr Palmer, he's a patient of Spencer's. I went to see him two days ago and he tore me off a strip for smoking – really laid into me about it he did. Said that it would lead me to an early grave and that I'd be stupid if I didn't give it up, and now I've just seen him get out of his car smoking himself. He stubbed it out when he got to the door. It's sheer hypocrisy, that is.'

'Perhaps he needed to smoke to calm his nerves because he's coming to see Spencer and it's probably a case of "do as I say, not as I do", Mrs Crossley.'

'Well I wouldn't mind but he made me feel like I must be a complete moron to even think about smoking and all the time he's smoking himself.'

'Do you smoke a lot?'

'Not that many.'

'How many?'

'I don't know; but not that many. Anyway I was reading an article in a magazine last week and it said that smoking's not as bad for you as many doctors think.'

'It can't be very good for you, I'm sure you'd be healthier if you didn't smoke and as for your doctor, why don't you transfer to Dr MacKean; I'm sure he'd be far more sympathetic.'

'Oh no, I used to go to him and he upset me well and truly by telling me I was overweight. You can imagine what I said about that – him telling me I'm overweight when he's a big fat lump himself.'

'Oh dear but I'm sure he had your best interests at heart.'

'Well he didn't have to be so rude about it. Medical people seem to think they're a law unto themselves – different from the rest of us. I bet you tell your patients not to eat sweets and then go and eat them yourself. Perhaps I am a bit overweight but there's a right way and a wrong way to tell someone. Anyway I was reading an article in a magazine yesterday which said that the finest things out to keep you fit and healthy are broccoli and beetroot so I'm going to start eating them.'

'I'm sure they're good for you but you can't believe everything you read in magazines, Mrs Crossley.'

'Well I'm going to give them a try anyway.'

I left Mrs Crossley still muttering to herself and I wondered if she would keep out of Dr Palmer's way or whether she would confront him and mention his smoking. I didn't wait to find out because Mr Rutherford senior was coming to have his teeth scaled. He arrived wearing the same frayed clothes he wore when he came with 'young Harold' and shuffled into my surgery grunting bad temperedly. I wondered whether I should enquire as to how his son was and whether he had come to terms with his inability to whistle the dog after I'd filled his front teeth. However I decided that it would be advisable to keep off the subject so I said to him, 'have you no quotation for me today?'

'*Under all speech that is good for anything there lies a silence that is better. Silence is deep as Eternity; speech is shallow as time.*'

145

'I knew you wouldn't disappoint me,' I commented, hoping that this quotation reflected the way he was feeling and that today he would be less vociferous and let me get on with the job in hand, which was scaling his teeth. Removing a lifetime's deposits of tartar was like chipping away at a lump of granite with a blunt penknife and I soon found myself wishing I had my new dental unit which would have a built-in ultrasonic scaler. Unfortunately I didn't, so I had to do the scaling with hand instruments which was extremely laborious and tiring. By the time I had finished, sweat was pouring from my brow and my wrist was aching terribly.

'Are you sure this is doing any good?' asked Mr Rutherford who was looking more than slightly perturbed by the amount of blood he was losing from his gums.

'It's the only way,' I assured him. 'Now it's up to you to prevent the tartar from reforming by brushing. I assume you bought a toothbrush?'

'Yes and I've brought it with me to prove it.'

He pulled out from his top pocket the most colossal toothbrush I had ever seen.

'Is that it?' I asked stupidly, staring in utter disbelief at the sheer size of it.

'Why yes,' he replied, sensing my lack of approval. 'What's wrong with it?'

'It's gigantic; it's more like a lavatory brush than a toothbrush. Where on earth did you get it from?'

'I got it from the local chemist. To start with I bought one from the supermarket but it was a silly little thing and was useless. As Jane Austen put it:-

The little bit of ivory on which I work with so fine a brush as produces little effect after much effort.

'I decided I needed a man-sized brush and the local chemist rummaged through his old stock and found me this one. He said he'd had it ages because nobody buys brushes like this anymore. It's also genuine bristle – not this nylon rubbish.'

'I'm sorry, Mr Rutherford but it's ridiculous; it's far too big to be any good. You'll never be able to clean your teeth properly with it. You need a brush with a small head so that you can reach every tooth.'

I looked closely at his huge brush and noted that the bristles were perfectly straight and in pristine condition. My immediate thought was that the brush had not been used. I eyed him suspiciously and put it to him, 'are you actually using it?'

'I am, I am but the trouble is when you've never been in the habit of cleaning your teeth, it isn't easy to remember. The other problem is that you told me to clean my teeth at bedtime and I usually take a nip of whisky to bed with me.'

'Why is that a problem?'

'Well after I've drained my glass I usually drop off to sleep. It makes me forget everything so I don't think about cleaning my teeth.'

'I see, but can't you clean your teeth before you drink the whisky?'

'What and spoil the flavour of my beautiful twelve year old Glenlivet with the fowl taste of toothpaste? I'm sorry but that really is asking too much. I'm prepared to make sacrifices to save my teeth but there are certain things that are quite out of the question and that's one of them. Why it's unthinkable.'

'What about in the mornings?'

'I've cleaned them most mornings; I may have forgotten once or twice. It's not easy to remember.'

'Well you really are going to have to try harder unless you want to lose your teeth. Now I'm going to show you how I want you to clean them.'

'You're what? Do you take me for a complete idiot? Show me how to brush my teeth at my age? This is kindergarten stuff. I may never have used a toothbrush but I'm not so stupid that I wouldn't know how to use one. I'm sorry my boy but I've got better things to do with my time than to sit here listening to you talking to me as if I'm a five year old. I'm going back to my gardening. Where's my stick?'

'Please, Mr Rutherford, wait a minute. Brushing your teeth is more difficult than you think. Few people do it properly.'

'No, I'm going.'

His mind appeared to be made up and it seemed there was nothing I could do to stop him leaving; then I had an idea.

'Would you let Wendy show you how to brush your teeth? You can go into the office with her – there's no-one else in there and she'll go through it with you.'

His face immediately lit up. 'I may be able to stay a few minutes longer provided it doesn't take too long. Where is the lovely girl?'

'I'll go and find her. Come with me to the office.'

I swear Mr Rutherford had a spring in his step at the prospect of rubbing shoulders with Wendy and I couldn't help thinking that there was still life in the old dog but I very much doubted whether her instructions would have any effect on him. It was never easy to change someone's habits of a lifetime and probably impossible in the case of someone as set in his ways as Mr Rutherford.

I had arranged to finish early that day so that I would have time to go to the dental supply company's showrooms to look at new equipment. My last patient was Mrs Newman who was coming to look at the temporary crowns we had made for her. They looked enormous on the plaster model and I couldn't believe they would look sensible in her mouth but the final decision would be made by her, not by me, and she had given clear instructions that this was what she wanted.

'They're perfect, Mr Derwent, exactly what I wanted.'

'You're sure they aren't too big, Mrs Newman? We have to be sure before we go ahead with the permanent crowns.'

'I'm absolutely sure; they look great.'

'In that case, we need to make an appointment so that I can prepare your teeth for the permanent crowns. There won't be a lot of tooth preparation necessary; I really just need to define the margins so that the edges of the crowns don't irritate your gums. Wendy will sort out an appointment for you.'

'Can't I just keep these?'

'I'm afraid not. They're only plastic and therefore not very strong. You'd soon break them and because your teeth have not been prepared they don't fit properly at gum level.'

'The permanent crowns will look as good as this, won't they and they won't be any smaller?'

'Same size, I promise and they'll look better because the technician will build in some "character" which the temporary crowns don't have.'

As soon as Mrs Newman had left, I set off for the showrooms of the Ashcroft Dental Supply Company. I was delighted that Spencer had agreed to let me re-equip my surgery. I found the equipment installed at present very inefficient and difficult to use. The setup had not been ergonomically designed and often things were simply in the wrong place for ease of operation. I had never really come to terms with the revolving stool arrangement that Spencer had invented, and of which he was so proud. Although I was more or less familiar with its idiosyncrasies, I could not share his enthusiasm for the design and I still felt very precariously balanced and unstable when I was on it. He was accustomed to working with his patient sitting upright but I wasn't. Although it was possible to tip the dental chair right back, I was unable to work on a patient in this position because the tubing on the drill wasn't long enough to allow it to reach the patient's mouth.

Spencer's claim that patients didn't like to lie flat for their treatment was true for some of them, particularly the older ones, but I found that it was very tiring to have to bend forward in order to see to the back of a patient's mouth, particularly for more complicated procedures when it was sometimes necessary to maintain this position for a long time. I was really looking forward to working with new equipment which would make life in the surgery much pleasanter and more efficient and I couldn't wait for the chance to go off to the dental supply company's premises where I could see what they had to offer.

Soon I was listening to the persuasive patter of an enthusiastic salesman who was as keen to sell as I was to buy. It was extremely difficult to make a decision because there was so much to choose from. I was expecting the choice to be far more restricted bearing in mind that there are relatively few dentists in the country and buying new equipment is not something they are likely to do very often, which means that the market must be fairly limited. It crossed my mind that if every dentist felt the same way as Spencer about new equipment, the manufacturers of dental equipment would all go out of business.

It was almost as if the salesman was able to read my thoughts.

'It may surprise you, Mr Derwent,' he explained encouragingly, 'but it is in fact, common practice for many dentists to buy complete new surgeries every five years or so. That way they can be sure they always have the very latest and there are considerable tax advantages in doing so.'

'Is that right?'

'Oh yes indeed, Mr Derwent. You need to discuss it with your accountant and he will advise you.'

I didn't like to tell him that I was merely an associate in Spencer's practice and that I didn't actually have an accountant but his words made me wonder if perhaps I ought to consult one. So far, the Inland Revenue had not contacted me and I hadn't paid any tax

149

on my earning yet, but I knew that this situation would almost certainly change very soon.

After looking at virtually everything on offer I eventually made up my mind as to what I liked best.

'That's a very good choice if I may say so, sir,' said the salesman in his most reassuring tone. 'I'm sure you'll find that it will give you many years of trouble-free service.'

It wasn't the cheapest but it wasn't the most expensive either, though the cost was still enough to make my eyes water. I didn't have that sort of money and I was going to have to borrow it from somewhere. The prospect of approaching my bank manager for a loan caused me a degree of apprehension but the salesman was able to cut short my anxiety.

'There are schemes in place which allow the cost to be spread over a period of time at very favourable rates of interest.'

'Really?' I sighed with relief. 'That would be very helpful.'

Before I had time to justify my impecunious state to the salesman, he continued. 'You would be foolish to pay for it outright, in fact, no-one does. It makes more sense to spread the cost over a period of several years. You could, of course, obtain a loan from your bank if you wish but I think you will find our interest rates very competitive.'

'In that case, I'll go with your scheme.'

'Very well, Mr Derwent, I'll make out a sales invoice and we'll fill in a finance form straight away, if you would like to.'

'Yes, let's do it,' I responded somewhat impulsively.

Without further ado, the necessary paperwork was completed and we shook hands on the deal.

'The cost includes installation provided that mains water, electricity and drainage are laid on to where the equipment will be installed and it's your responsibility to arrange that. We'll do the rest. When would you like us to install it?'

'I can't say at this moment. The room in which it's to be installed has to be cleared and possibly decorated and the services have to be put in.'

'That's no problem at all, Mr Derwent. We'll look after the equipment for you until you're ready for it. Just let us know when you want us to deliver it.'

I felt very excited as I drove back to the surgery and I wondered how I was going to persuade Spencer to get on with the job of clearing his sitting room. He had worked very quickly to set up the new waiting room and in moving his surgery downstairs but his speediness was uncharacteristic and I had a strong feeling that the next stage of the practice reorganization was going to proceed much more slowly. I didn't want him to think I was harassing him but now that I had ordered my new equipment I was naturally anxious to start using it as soon as possible.

'I've ordered my new equipment, Spencer.'

'Already? You didn't waste any time, did you? Are you sure you've chosen wisely because you couldn't possibly have surveyed the whole market in such a short time?'

'I went to Ashcroft Dental Supply Company's showrooms and looked at everything they have on offer. They have a lot to choose from.'

'I know they do, Justin, but they aren't the only dental supply company. There are lots of others. You might have done better elsewhere.'

'You could go on looking for ever but I went to the local company because they will deliver and install which might be a problem if I bought from further afield. Anyway, I think they had a wide range and I'm happy with what I've chosen.'

'That's all that matters then,' said Spencer dismissively.

'The unit I've chosen is really streamlined with two high speed drill outlets, a high-torque air motor, ultrasonic scaler, a very bright operating light, and it has a built in aspirator like the one you've just acquired.'

'Really?' replied Spencer with about as much enthusiasm as if he'd just discovered he had lost heavily on the stock market. 'All I can say is that I hope it isn't as unreliable as modern cars, but if it's what you want, Justin, who am I to criticise? As you are well aware, I think it's a terrible waste of money but the dental companies must sell it or they wouldn't keep making it.'

'Apparently, some dentists replace the whole lot every five years or so.'

'That's because it's so badly made it won't last any longer than that.'

I am quite sure that I failed to convince him that the new equipment would have significant advantages over the equipment I was using at present. In the end I decided I might as well save my breath, as my words were falling on deaf ears but I couldn't help

151

trying to ascertain from him when I would be able to get the dental company to install it.

'You'll appreciate that I'm anxious to start using it as soon as possible, Spencer, so I would be very, very grateful if you'll clear the sitting room soon.'

'I'll get on with it as soon as possible, Justin,' was all he would say, which was a source of great frustration.

Each morning when I arrived for work I would poke my nose into his sitting room to see if there was any evidence that he was beginning to move out his furniture but after a week there was still no sign of activity. He was now working in his downstairs surgery and as far as he was concerned the problem of getting patients like Lady Gascoyne-Fairley upstairs had been resolved. He had assured me that he wanted to complete the reorganization as quickly as possible which included moving me and the office downstairs but so far there was no indication that he intended to proceed with the final phase of the move in the immediate future and I was beginning to get impatient.

CHAPTER TWENTY THREE

I had started to realize that I wasn't looking after myself very well when it came to meals. Making do with something quick and easy rather than nutritious had become something of a habit and I had made a resolution to change my ways. I firmly believed that a well-balanced diet was a recipe for good health so it made sense to take a little bit of extra trouble to make sure I followed that philosophy. As I served my grilled plaice garnished with broad leafed parsley and a slice of lemon and accompanied with fresh salad and whole meal bread I thought how appetizing it looked and I eagerly sat down to enjoy it. It wasn't exactly cordon bleu but it was a vast improvement on the beans and scrambled eggs which had become my staple diet in recent weeks. I had only sampled one delicious mouthful when, much to my annoyance, the telephone rang.

Why did it have to ring at that moment? I considered letting it ring but then I thought it might be something important so I resigned myself to having my meal interrupted, but as I picked up the receiver, I fully intended to get rid of the caller as quickly as possible.

'Hello, Justin, it's Harriet Brooks here. Do you remember me?'

'Hello, Harriet. Of course I remember you. How are you?'

'I'm very well, thank you, Justin. I hope you don't mind my phoning you at home; I phoned your surgery and spoke to Mr Padginton who said you'd already left but he felt sure you wouldn't mind if I phoned you at home and he gave me your number.'

'Of course I don't mind; it's lovely to hear from you. What can I do for you?'

'You remember that I'm studying psychology? Well I'm doing a research project on the effects of stress and apprehension on a person's behaviour and it occurred to me that you must witness these effects every day because most people find visiting the dentist very stressful. I wondered if you would be prepared to help me with this project.'

'I'd be very happy to help if you think I can be of use to you. What do you want me to do?'

'I was wondering if you could perhaps spare me half an hour after work one day so that I could talk to you about it; I don't want to take up too much of your time but if you could spend a few minutes I'm sure your experience would be most informative.'

'When did you start the project? Have you got very far with it?'

'No, I've only just started. My tutor said we had to come up with ideas for research projects and it was only after I came to see you that it occurred to me this might be a good subject.'

'I suppose I tend to forget that people are nervous when they come to see me but I expect many of them are, if I think about it.'

'I'm sure they are,' said Harriet, 'and it's understandable that you tend to forget because it's quite normal to be nervous and because it's so common, you don't notice it any more. What I'm really concerned about is that very often you will be giving out important advice and information and the fact that they are nervous will affect their ability to take in this information.'

'We have found it's advisable to give information in writing because otherwise it tends to get ignored.'

'Exactly, and part of my research is to try and establish to what extent one's ability to assimilate information is impaired due to stress or anxiety. Anyway, will you help me with the project if I come to your surgery one day after work?'

'Of course I will, Harriet, I'll be delighted to help. Why don't you let me take you out for a drink one evening then we'll have more time?'

'Won't your girlfriend object if you take me out for a drink?'

'I haven't really got a girlfriend.'

'Are you sure, Justin? I thought I saw you with someone last weekend and let's just say that I got the impression she was your girlfriend.'

'I think I know what you're referring to. It's true I've been out with someone a few times but it isn't serious, not as far as I'm concerned anyway.'

'Perhaps she sees it differently?'

'Perhaps she does but I can assure you the relationship isn't really going anywhere. I would like to take you out for a drink, Harriet, if you'll let me.'

The prospect of taking Harriet out convinced me immediately that Sarah and I really didn't have a long-term future together. I had had my doubts about it previously but now my mind was absolutely clear. When I said to Harriet that the relationship wasn't going anywhere, I was speaking the absolute truth. I hadn't been completely sure about it until that moment but now I was.

'I would like it too, Justin, but I wouldn't want to cause any trouble between you and your …err …friend. I'm prepared to meet you at your surgery if it would be easier.'

'I really would like to take you out, Harriet. Your project sounds very interesting and it would be much better to discuss it over a drink in a pub somewhere. It's not that I don't like my work but I prefer to get away from the surgery as soon as I can after a long day.'

'I can understand that and I would love to go out with you if you are absolutely sure it won't cause any trouble.'

'I'm sure.'

I was about to suggest taking her out on Saturday evening but then I remembered that I had arranged to meet Sarah.

'Would Friday evening suit you?'

'Friday would be fine.'

'Good, then I'll pick you up at eight o'clock.'

'Will you come to my house?'

'Yes, of course.'

'Then I'd better give you my address.'

I already knew where she lived because I had made a mental note of her address from her dental record card. I was on the point of telling her I knew; then I thought better of it.

'Yes, of course and if you give me your telephone number I can phone if I need to contact you. Wait a second whilst I get a pen and some paper.'

After I put down the phone, my elation at the opportunity to see Harriet again after I had thought she had disappeared from my life forever completely overshadowed my enthusiasm for my grilled plaice. I couldn't believe she had telephoned me and I found myself wondering if she was actually interested in me and in fact, the project was just an excuse to contact me. But then I wrote off the idea deciding that it was merely wishful thinking on my part. My biggest problem now was Sarah. Harriet was aware of her presence and I had deliberately played down the relationship to the point where I wasn't sure I had been entirely honest, but what else could I have done? I felt sure I would want to go on seeing Harriet if she was willing but I couldn't do so without telling Sarah. I'm sure Richard Darcy wouldn't have considered this to be much of a problem – he frequently moved from one woman to the next without any apparent difficulty but I didn't have his experience.

For some reason I couldn't wait to tell Wendy that Harriet had phoned me and that I was going to take her out for a drink.

'So you're two-timing, Justin. Be very careful because you can finish up losing both of them.'

'I know that from previous experience though I didn't lose them completely. Sarah was one of them and she's still on the scene and that's the trouble.'

'But if you allowed her to come back into your life, you must like her.'

'Yes I do, but I think I like Harriet more.'

'You don't really know enough about her at this stage, but I knew you were attracted to her from the start. I said this to you, didn't I?'

'Yes you did, Wendy, and you were right – I'm attracted to her very much. I don't know why but there's just something about her that appeals to me in a way that I've never experienced before.'

'Well I hope it all works out for you, Justin, but I'm just saying that you should tread very carefully and before you tell Sarah, be absolutely sure you want to finish with her because I can't believe she'll give you another chance.'

CHAPTER TWENTY FOUR

The week seemed to pass unbearably slowly. My excitement at the prospect of taking Harriet out was gradually replaced by apprehension as Friday loomed nearer. At the back of my mind was the realization that I was going out with her because she had asked me to help with her research project which wasn't quite the same as taking her out on a date, whereby the reason for our coming together would have been that we wanted to share each other's company. I could not deny that this was my reason for wanting to see her; the question was: how did she feel about it?

My palms felt clammy against the steering wheel as I turned into the road where she lived. I drove slowly looking at the house numbers as I went by, searching for number 88, but I needn't have bothered because Harriet was standing outside the freshly painted white gate of her house. Had I been looking ahead I would have seen her immediately, as her crisp, white linen trouser suit and auburn hair stood out in marked contrast against a dark green background formed by a well-manicured privet hedge. She looked young, fresh and vibrant in the evening sun and waved when she saw my car which, for some reason, made me feel slightly less anxious.

'Thank you so much for agreeing to see me,' was her opening statement as she slid on to my gleaming leather passenger seat, which had been meticulously scoured to remove all traces of dust and grime prior to my leaving home. Although she spoke with obvious gratitude, her words had a ring of formality and made me feel like a business associate who had offered to meet with her in order to advise on a commercial venture she was contemplating.

'The pleasure's all mine,' I replied, desperately trying to think how I could subtly get across the message that I had arranged to meet her because I really wanted to and not because I was merely answering her request for assistance with her project.

'You didn't have to take me out, Justin, I would have been happy to come to your surgery. I know you're busy.'

This announcement further shattered my confidence. I felt even more convinced that her objective was solely to pick my brains and the harsh possibility that there was no other reason for her being with me, poured down on me like a cold shower.

We stopped at some traffic lights and I took the opportunity to look straight into her crystal-clear blue eyes and vainly struggled to convey my feelings to her.

'I'm delighted to take you out, Harriet. I really enjoyed talking to you in the supermarket and I hoped we might get the chance to meet again so I was pleased when you phoned me.'

'I enjoyed talking to you and I too, hoped we might meet again. I would have phoned you sooner about my project but when I saw you with someone who appeared to be your girlfriend I thought perhaps I shouldn't.'

'I've told you; she isn't really my girlfriend.'

'I did see you kissing, so it was a reasonable assumption that she was someone special. Anyway, it put me off phoning you but then I thought there was no harm in meeting you at your surgery and I felt sure you wouldn't mind helping me with my project.'

'Of course I don't mind; I hope I can give you some useful information.'

'If the girl I saw you kissing isn't your girlfriend, what is your relationship? You can understand why I thought she was your girlfriend, can't you? It was such a shock; I nearly drove into a lamp post.'

'I know you did. Sarah was very disparaging about your driving and it made me think about your encounter with the petrol pumps.' I smiled at the recollection.

'It wasn't funny, Justin.'

'I know and I don't mean to laugh. As for Sarah, I've been out with her two or three times that's all and it isn't serious. Honestly, Harriet.'

A twinge of guilt hit me as I remembered I was due to see Sarah tomorrow evening but I decided it was probably best not to tell Harriet. I thought I would try to change the subject.

'Anyway, let's talk about you. How are your studies going?'

'I'm supposed to be preparing for my finals now so I ought to be working hard but I'm finding it difficult to put my mind to it.'

'Too many distractions, I imagine. Do you have a boyfriend?'

'Not really. There are lots of boys at university and we all go out together as a mixed group but there isn't anyone special.'

'I'm surprised – a lovely girl like you.'

Harriet ignored the compliment.

'Have you had a good week?' I enquired, anxious to keep the conversation flowing but off the subject of Sarah.

'Not really. You remember my telling you I was taking a teaching certificate? Well I was sent to a large mixed comprehensive school on teaching practice this week and what do you think they got me to teach?'

'I've no idea.'

'Sex education!'

'No!'

'They did! It was awful.'

'How old were the pupils?'

'Sixteen and I can tell you; most of them know a good deal more about it than I do. It was so embarrassing.'

'I can imagine. It was very unfair of the school to put you in that position. Poor you, but at least you got through it and it's over now.'

'No it isn't. I got through it but that was only the first lesson. The second instalment is due to follow next week and a third the week after.'

'My God! I don't envy you having to do that.'

Although Harriet was understandably troubled and uncomfortable about the situation she had been thrown into she was nevertheless able to see the funny side of it. Laughing about it together helped to melt the ice between us and soon I felt much more relaxed.

We stopped off at a quiet little country pub and spent a thoroughly enjoyable couple of hours chatting away about all sorts of different subjects. We discussed her project for some of the time but it did not dominate the conversation and by the time we left I was beginning to think that maybe she was interested in me as a person rather than merely as someone who could supply her with information to assist with her studies.

The sky was clear and there was a full moon looking down on us as I drove deliberately slowly back in the direction of Luccombury. The longer I spent in Harriet's company the more I became captivated by her and I had no intention of hastening the journey home. She was bright, had a good sense of humour, and was able to talk intelligently about any subject you cared to mention as well as being overwhelmingly attractive.

'Would you like to come back to my cottage for coffee?' I ventured. 'It isn't very late.'

I was amazed and delighted when she accepted and it was noticeable that our rate of travel suddenly increased dramatically as my right foot no longer seemed reluctant to apply pressure to the accelerator pedal.

'It's a lovely little cottage,' Harriet enthused as the characterful sitting room became bathed in light from the table lamp, which I had chosen to switch on in preference to the harsher, less romantic wall lights. 'How long have you lived here?'

'Ever since I came to Luccombury. I was lucky enough to find it during my first week here. I don't own it, unfortunately; I only rent it but it suits me just fine.'

Harriet made herself comfortable on the sofa and I went to make some coffee. We chatted and I switched on the record player though we kept the volume deliberately low because conversation, which was now flowing freely and easily, was the most important feature of our evening together. Neither of us wanted the music to be overpowering.

I was about to make a second pot of coffee when there was a loud knock on the door. My heart sank and my first thought was that it might be Sarah. Perhaps she had seen Harriet and me out together, perhaps she had even followed me to find out what I was up to. I prayed it wouldn't be her because that would undoubtedly ruin what up to now had been a splendid evening. I could feel the colour drain from my face as I shuffled to the door.

'Sorry to disturb 'ee, Justin. I've been waiting for 'ee to come back.'

At first, relief swept over me when I saw Ephraim standing at the door but his presence was not particularly welcome at that moment either. However, before I could tell him to go away or think of any other excuse for not inviting him in, he and a very grubby looking Nellie pushed their way past me.

'I've been back some time, Ephraim.' I said wondering why he had waited nearly an hour before knocking on my door.

'I know and I wasn't goin' to trouble 'ee 'cos I saw the young lady like but I 'ad to come as I'm in trouble.'

Nellie shot straight over to where Harriet was sitting and was already enjoying the attention Harriet was giving her. It was quite clear that Harriet loved dogs and didn't seem to be the slightest bit concerned that Nellie looked as if she had just walked through a field of mud. I introduced Harriet to Ephraim and the two of them shook hands. I noticed that Ephraim was courteous enough to wipe his hand down the side of his trousers before offering it to Harriet though the action probably deposited more dirt than it removed.

'So what's the trouble, Epraim?'

He looked very shifty and hesitated for some considerable time as if trying to pluck up courage to make his announcement. Finally, in a shameful whisper he uttered, 'I've got toothache.'

'How long have you had it?'

'On and off for the best part of a month.'

'And I suppose it's really bad now?'

'Aye 'tis that, Justin, I've been bangin' my head against the wall all evening. My jaw's swollen now an' all.'

'Have you taken anything for it – pain killers?'

'I took some aspirin that I 'ad lying in a drawer but they didn't do no good. Per'aps they've lost their strength a bit – I've 'ad 'em a long time.'

'How long?'

'I don't rightly know but years, in fact come to think of it, must be over twenty years.'

'Then I suspect they have lost their strength but if your jaw is swollen it sounds as if you've got an abscess and you need antibiotics.'

'I think I might 'ave some o' they but I didn't think to take 'em. Will they do some good?'

'Depends what they are and how long you've had them.'

'Not that long. Vet gave 'em to Nellie 'cos she 'ad an infected paw but I only gave 'er a couple and her paw got better so I kept the rest thinkin' they might come in 'andy one day. I never thought to take they for this toothache.'

'I wouldn't recommend you take Nellie's tablets. I've no idea what vets give to dogs to treat infection – they might not be safe for humans.'

'He said they were antibiotics. Antibiotics are antibiotics, aren't they?'

Out of the corner of my eye I could see Harriet trying to keep a straight face as she continued to stroke Nellie. 'There are different types of antibiotics which are designed to be active against the particular bacteria causing the infection. Nellie's antibiotics might be the wrong type even if they aren't actually harmful. I can't do anything for you tonight but first thing tomorrow morning I'll go to the surgery and write a prescription. In the meantime, I can give you some paracetamol tablets which might help ease the pain.'

'That be real kind, Justin.'

'You'd better let me have a look at the tooth that's causing the trouble.'

'Does 'ee 'ave to? If I take the tablets they should sort it out and that'll be the end of it, won't it?'

'I'm afraid not, Ephraim. The antibiotics will help control the infection and take down the swelling but when you stop taking them the problem will recur unless you have the tooth removed.'

I watched the colour drain from his face just as it had drained from mine when I thought it might be Sarah at the door.

'Ooh, I don't think 'twill be necessary to take it out, Justin, will it?' His tone was not merely quizzical; there was a strong element of pleading in his voice.

'Open your mouth and let me see the tooth.'

Very reluctantly, Ephraim walked over to me and half-heartedly opened his mouth and pointed to the bottom left side.

'You'll need to open wider than that, Ephraim. I can't see anything.'

Very grudgingly he stretched his mouth only fractionally wider, but it was enough to confirm what I had suspected. It was not a pretty sight as virtually every tooth was broken off at gum level and all that was left was a row of black stumps. However I was able to see that the gum around one particular stump was red, inflamed and swollen. That one had to be the offending premolar but it wasn't the only tooth that needed extracting. I decided, however, that now was not a good time to start talking about multiple extractions.

'It'll have to come out, Ephraim; it's badly infected and isn't doing your general health any good.'

'There ain't nothin' wrong with my health – I've just got toothache that's all. It'll settle down if you give me the right tablets.'

'If I didn't know better, I'd say you were scared to have it out.'

162

'What me scared? Of 'avin' a tooth out? Don't make me laugh.' I glanced at Harriet who was still making a fuss of Nellie and finding the whole episode highly amusing but she didn't say anything.

'All right then, I'll get you some tablets first thing tomorrow and I'll make an appointment for you later in the week when it's calmed down a bit and I'll extract it.'

'I ain't at all sure I can manage next week, Justin; I've a lot on.'

'Really, Ephraim. I promise it won't take very long. Surely you can spare me half an hour out of your busy week. I suggest you go home now and take two of these paracetamol tablets and I'll get you a prescription for antibiotics first thing tomorrow.'

Ephraim trundled off into the night holding the left side of his jaw and looking extremely worried. Nellie followed faithfully.

'Do you think he'll let you extract his tooth, Justin?' asked Harriet as I re-joined her on the sofa.

'It'll be a minor miracle if he does; he's obviously terrified but he'll probably be forced to have it out eventually because it's almost certain to flare up again at some stage. The antibiotics will help for a while but they won't cure it though I do think his behaviour will probably provide useful information for your research project.'

'That's true, Justin, I hope you'll be watching him closely and making notes on my behalf.'

'I'll do my best, Harriet. Now I'll get us that coffee.'

I found a packet of ginger nuts to accompany the coffee and we munched away quite happily, oblivious to the fact that it was now getting late. Harriet didn't seem in any hurry to leave and I was more than happy to let her stay as long as she wanted. We were both startled when the telephone rang and I wondered who could possibly be phoning me at that time of night.

'Is that Mr Derwent?' said the female on the line.

'It is.'

'Do you have someone called Harriet there with you?'

'Yes I do. Who's calling?'

'It's her mother. I'm getting a bit worried about her because it's getting very late.'

'I can assure you she's perfectly all right. Would you like to speak to her?'

Harriet didn't look at all pleased as she took the phone from me. 'Why on earth are you phoning, mother? I'm all right. Yes, yes.

163

No I shall be home soon, now go to bed and stop worrying.' She replaced the handset and raised her eyes. Her expression suggested she was feeling exasperation and embarrassment.

'I'm sorry, Justin. I don't know how she managed to get hold of your phone number. She treats me like a five-year-old at times – it's so humiliating.'

'She's obviously concerned about you so don't be too hard on her. Anyway, I'd better take you home now.'

'My goodness, is that the time? I must admit I didn't realise it was as late as that. I'm sorry if I've kept you up.'

'You haven't, Harriet. It's been a lovely evening and I've really enjoyed your company.'

'I've enjoyed it too, very much.'

'I'd like to see you again.'

'That would be nice, Justin.'

We were standing facing each other and I felt myself being drawn towards her. It seemed the most natural thing in the world to kiss her and somehow I got the impression she wouldn't have objected if I had, but my courage failed me. I was worried that I was reading the signs wrongly and the last thing I wanted was to upset her by overstepping the mark. I got the notion she had had a sheltered upbringing by a mother who was highly protective so I decided I ought to take things very slowly. The other nagging thought was that Sarah was still on the scene and I knew from past experience that life could become very complicated if you started to impinge on the emotions of two women at the same time.

I wanted to make arrangements to see Harriet again there and then but at the moment I felt I needed to tread carefully.

'I'll give you a ring sometime, if I may,' I said to her somewhat vaguely. As I said it I thought it didn't sound as though I was all that enthusiastic which was certainly not the sentiment I wanted to convey.

'I'll look forward to it,' she replied.

CHAPTER TWENTY FIVE

I was up early next morning in spite of having had a late night. Immediately after breakfast I went to the surgery and wrote a prescription for amoxicillin for Ephraim. I decided I would call in at the pharmacist's on my way back to get the tablets as it occurred to me that he might not appreciate it was important for him to start taking them as soon as possible. In fact, I thought that there was a chance he might not bother to get them at all, especially if the paracetamol I had given him had succeeded in easing the pain.

When I got back to his cottage he opened the door to me looking extremely sorry for himself. His face was now visibly swollen and his eyes were red, which told me that he had not slept very well.

' 'tis bad, Justin,' were his first words but he didn't have to say it; I knew as soon as I saw him.

'I suggest you take two of these immediately; another one this afternoon and one before you go to bed tonight.'

'Will they stop the pain? I'm in agony.'

'Not straightaway, the pain will ease when the swelling goes down. You'll need painkillers for a day or two at least. Did the ones I gave you do any good?'

'No – didn't touch it. I'll need something stronger. Can you give me some?'

'You'll need another prescription. If I'd known I'd have got you some; I'll have to go back to the surgery later this morning, if you can hang on.'

'I've drunk near on a bottle o' whisky to try an' deaden it.'

'In that case, I'll have to go and get them for you. You can't possibly drive.'

'I've drunk this much an' driven before.'

I knew that Ephraim's driving was pretty reckless at the best of times; I dreaded to think what it would be like after that much alcohol. 'No, you stay here. I'll get the painkillers for you. Now let me have another look at your tooth. If the swelling's localized I might be able to incise it and release the pus. That would give you instant relief.'

'Incise it? You mean stick a knife in it?'

'Yes, that's right. If we drain off the pus it will feel a lot better.'

'I don't think I likes the sound o' that, Justin. Can't we just wait for the pills to work?'

'We can but it will take much longer.'

'I'll wait.'

'If you start the antibiotics now and don't forget to take them, they should bring the infection under control within a few days. I'll check with you each evening and as soon as they've worked I'll book you in to have the tooth extracted.'

'I don't know, Justin. As I said, I'm very busy this coming week.'

'Doing what?'

'This and that.'

'Well nothing is as important as getting this tooth sorted out. You can die of septicaemia from an infected tooth, you know.'

'Now you're scaring me, Justin. It's not very likely, is it?'

'Not very, but it can happen so I wouldn't ignore it if I were you.'

Ephraim fell very silent and his look of anguish intensified. I don't really think he believed me when I told him the condition could prove fatal and as it was extremely unlikely that this would happen I didn't really feel that I could labour the point. In any event, I felt sure the fear of having the tooth extracted outweighed his fear of dying. He took the tablets from me and retreated indoors whilst Nellie looked up at him with big brown soulful eyes, clearly concerned that her master was under the weather.

I got Ephraim his painkillers later in the morning and spent the rest of the day tidying up my cottage and polishing my car. I kept thinking about Harriet and how much I had enjoyed our evening together. For some reason I had felt apprehensive before I went to meet her but that was nothing compared with how I felt now as I set out to pick up Sarah. I didn't want to deceive her and I knew I ought to tell her about Harriet but I felt sure she wouldn't be very happy about it and I hated upsetting anyone, particularly people I liked. As I reflected on my evening with Harriet I started to have doubts as to how she felt. I was fairly sure she liked being with me and maybe she wanted us to go on seeing each other but then I found myself thinking that perhaps she was just a very pleasant, friendly girl whose feelings could easily be misconstrued and our meeting had been no more than a get together to discuss her project. Perhaps that's all there was to it and wishful thinking on my part had allowed me to build up hope that was not really justified. We hadn't kissed or held hands so what reason did I have for believing she was anything more than just a new friend and that's as far as it would go? Was there really any need to say anything to Sarah at this stage? Possibly the best course of action would be to wait and see if anything developed between me and Harriet before coming out into the open.

If I told Sarah, I felt sure she would say she didn't want to see me anymore and I doubted if she would be prepared to go along with the 'can't we still be friends?' request. I was very fond of her but if my meeting Harriet had achieved anything it was to convince me that my feelings for Sarah didn't go deep enough for our relationship to survive in the long term. I began to hope she might decide she wanted to end our association but that seemed unlikely at the present time, and if she didn't, then one day I would have to tell her that we didn't have a future together, which I would find difficult. The more I thought about it the more undecided I became as to what I should do at the present time and my mind went into a complete turmoil. In the end I took the coward's way out and decided not to say anything to Sarah about Harriet. If I went out with Harriet again and things began to develop between us then that would be the time to tell Sarah. Until then, I would say nothing.

I received the usual warm greeting from Sarah and her dogs when I presented myself at her door at eight o'clock as arranged and my conscience started to prick me that I was being unfair to her by not telling her about Harriet. I tried to dismiss the thought from my mind on the basis that I had analyzed the situation and chosen a course of action. Now I had to stick to it.

As it turned out, Sarah had received a phone call from some of her friends asking if we wanted to join them for drinks at a nearby pub and Sarah had accepted the invitation. From my point of view, this made things somewhat easier as we became involved in general conversation with other people. It also meant that I was spared having to make any promises regarding the parachute jump Sarah wanted us to engage in together, as mercifully, the subject was not raised.

When I took her home at the end of the evening I declined her invitation to go in for coffee on the grounds that I felt tired because I had had a late night the previous evening though I wasn't entirely honest as to why it had been late. I said that Ephraim had come to see me because he had toothache, which was truthful as far as it went. I deliberately refrained from making a definite arrangement to see Sarah again and told her I would telephone her sometime during the week. I don't think she was entirely happy with the arrangement and would have much preferred to pin me down to a particular day but she had come to accept that vague promises with a strong element of elusiveness was the way I tended to operate. Surprisingly, it didn't seem to occur to her that this tendency might equate with uncertainty about my feelings for her; or perhaps it did occur to her, but she chose to disregard it at this stage in our relationship.

CHAPTER TWENTY SIX

I was overjoyed by what I saw when I looked into Spencer's sitting room at the start of another working week. There were definite signs that the room was being cleared and the first steps towards my new surgery had been taken by Spencer over the weekend. They may only have been small, tentative steps but at least there was some progress being made at last.

'I've made a start, you'll be pleased to see, Justin,' he called out to me from the door of his surgery across the hall. I didn't know he was there and for a moment he startled me.

'So I see, Spencer. I can't tell you how pleased I am. You know how keen I am to get my new equipment installed. How long do you think it will take before I can get the plumbing and electrics set up in there?'

'Not long. In fact you don't need to wait until the room is completely clear. It may take a while for me to move out all the furniture but if I lift the carpet and clear the middle of the room you can get started. Have you decided where you're putting the chair?'

'I thought I'd put it roughly where that table is, facing the window. What do you think?

'It's entirely up to you, Justin. I'm sure you'll have planned it out to get the best arrangement. Anyway, I'm glad I caught you because I wanted to have a word with you about the son of one of my friends in the Sports Car Club. I've met the lad a few times at some of our race meetings and frankly I'm not very impressed; he seems far too confident for his own good. His father is a great chap who I get on with extremely well but his son is completely different. It appears that he's suddenly decided he might go into dentistry, though I don't attach too much importance to this because he changes his mind more often than I change my shirt. Last time I saw him he wanted to become an accountant like his father – no, I tell a lie – a stockbroker. It was the previous time I saw him he wanted to be an accountant. Well now he thinks dentistry is the best career for him and he's asked if he could come and sit in with us for a few days to get a feel of it. My heart sank when he asked me and the thought of him breathing down my neck whilst I'm trying to treat patients wasn't at all appealing. But then I thought that as you are nearer to his age maybe you'd quite like the idea of demonstrating your skills to him. You're at the forefront of the latest dental technology and will be able to answer any of his questions. Would you be prepared to let him sit in with you for a day or two?'

'I wouldn't mind.'

'That's great, Justin. I knew I could rely on you. I didn't really feel I could refuse but I'm sure he'll be better with you than he would be with me. He's arriving tomorrow about mid-morning.'

'How old is he?'

'Seventeen, I think, but going on fifty if you see what I mean.'

'I'll try to sell dentistry to him as best I can.'

'I wouldn't try too hard. Dentistry might well be better off without him. Just carry on as normal, let him watch, and answer his questions. Might be a good idea to line up a juicy extraction or two – that should help him decide whether or not he has the stomach for the job.' With a slightly sadistic glint in his eye he retreated to his surgery and left me gazing into his sitting room. I tried to visualize my new equipment fully installed and the room re-decorated; I felt sure it would look impressive to patients and I was becoming very impatient to get on with it. At least Spencer had made a start on the room so things were beginning to move along. It simply wasn't happening quickly enough for me.

Next morning when I arrived at the practice I once again stuck my head into the room and much to my delight and surprise; I saw that the carpet had been rolled back so the floor area where I had indicated to Spencer that I wanted to site the chair was now clear. That meant I could go ahead and arrange for plumbing and electricity to be installed. Another twinge of excitement shot through me as I could see my objective move one step nearer to fruition.

I thought I'd start the day with a cup of coffee and I went into the kitchen just in time to see Mrs Crossley slump back into a chair with a look of abject terror on her face. She was clutching a weighty medical textbook she had taken from Spencer's bookshelf and I witnessed the last trace of colour drain from her usually ruddy complexion. She groaned in utter despair and I thought she was about to pass out.

'What on earth's the matter, Mrs Crossley? You look as white as a sheet.'

'It's the worst,' she sobbed, 'the big "C", there's no doubt about it; it says so here.'

'What are you talking about?'

'I've got cancer.'

I looked again at the book in her trembling hand and realized that, apart from anything else that might be afflicting her; she was definitely suffering from a severe attack of self-diagnosis.

'You don't know you've got cancer. Have you seen a doctor?'

'I don't need to. I've got all the symptoms, they're all set out here and I've got them; especially the blood.'

'You're bleeding from somewhere you shouldn't be, are you?'

'Ahh, dreadfully.'

'When did it start?'

'Only recently but it's really bad.'

'Can I ask where you're bleeding?' I ventured falteringly, not wishing to offend or embarrass her.

Mrs Crossley opened her mouth to speak but no sound came out and she waved a finger up and down pointing to somewhere below her waist.

'Is it in your urine?' I enquired trying to sound as clinical and detached as I could.

There was no reply; just sobbing, panting and a shake of the head then I spotted the title on the page she was referring to in the textbook and saw that she was reading about gastro-enterology.

'You think you've got bowel cancer, don't you?' I exclaimed.

'I don't think: I know,' she howled.

'You don't know; you're just guessing. It's not a good idea to read medical books because you can convince yourself you're suffering from all sorts of things. It's probably nothing at all to worry about but you really need to see your doctor as soon as possible. He'll be very understanding and the sooner it's attended to the better. Go and phone him now and make an appointment to see him.'

'I can't I'm too scared.'

'Then I'll get Wendy to do it for you.'

I went to find her, leaving poor Mrs Crossley looking absolutely panic-stricken and still seeking answers within the book.

Wendy went to look up Mrs Crossley's doctor's telephone number and reminded me that the son of Spencer's friend would be coming to sit in with me sometime during the morning. I had temporarily forgotten about him and although Spencer was very lukewarm to the idea of having a student in the surgery with him, I thought it might be quite enjoyable to show off my skills to a young man who was thinking of embarking on a career in dentistry. I wanted to try and make the experience interesting and informative and I scanned through my appointments for the day to see who was booked in and what treatments and techniques I would be able to demonstrate. It was fairly mixed; which was good. There was a patient for fillings, one for impressions for a denture, an extraction and a root filling as well as some check-ups.

I was taking a short coffee break when Hubert arrived. He was lankiness personified with dark brown eyes, black wavy hair and a prominent nose, chin and Adam's apple. I immediately noticed that his eyebrows met in the middle – a feature my mother said should always be viewed with suspicion as she claimed it was usually an indication of deceitfulness.

Spencer led him through the door and he greeted me with, 'Hi, Justin,' which although affable enough, seemed slightly over-familiar for someone of his age who I had never met before. Thinking back to when I was seventeen, I feel sure I would have been a little bit apprehensive and somewhat reserved in this sort of situation but Hubert showed no signs of any inhibitions whatsoever. We shook hands and I introduced him to Wendy. He beamed at her and for the next few minutes he didn't take his eyes off her for an instant, as if totally entranced by her. She completely ignored his penetrating gaze and carried on with her work as if he weren't present. As soon as she left the room he turned to me. 'How is it you dentists always employ such gorgeous-looking nurses? Where do you find them? Every dental nurse I've ever seen has always been an absolute knockout – except for Spencer's, of course.'

'That's not very nice, Hubert. Beryl is a very nice person and an excellent dental nurse. She might be a bit older than most but experience counts for a lot and she's extremely good with the patients.'

172

'So she might be but if you're going to be cooped up with someone all day and every day you want it to be someone good to look at.'

'You're supposed to give your attention to the patient, not your nurse – she's there to help you with your work.'

'Maybe but it must make life more pleasant if she's good-looking.'

I decided to divert attention to the practice of dentistry. 'So why have you decided that you'd like to become a dentist?'

'I haven't decided definitely – I'm considering it as a strong possibility – mainly because it's so well paid.'

'Is it?' I retorted in a tone which suggested that I viewed his opinion with scepticism.

'Oh, definitely,' said Hubert, 'particularly in the early years after qualification. I've done some research on it and in most jobs it takes several, sometimes many years before you start to earn big money whereas in dentistry you can start to rake it in immediately after qualifying. It might take a year or two to gather speed and efficiency but in no time at all you're one of the top earners in the country.'

'Is that so?'

'Yes it is. I've looked into it pretty carefully.'

'It's a demanding job though both physically and mentally. I think there are jobs in finance, for example, that aren't so physically demanding. It seems to me that many of the people in these jobs just shuffle bits of paper around and as long as they shuffle wisely the money comes in. With dentistry you have to earn every penny by physical effort and if you aren't actually carrying out treatment on a patient you aren't earning anything. Also, as you get older you can't work so quickly or for such long hours so your earnings diminish whilst in most other jobs your earnings go on rising throughout your career.'

'Yes but the great thing about dentistry is that you earn big money whilst you're young enough to enjoy it. There's no point in being rich when you're old and decrepit. You can always switch to something else when you're past it for dentistry.'

'Like what? It's not that easy to switch career especially later in life.'

'There's always something else you can do, like playing with stocks and shares. It can be risky so I wouldn't want to do it as a

173

career from the start but it's something worth thinking about later on in life.'

'You seem to have thought about it very thoroughly but I'm not sure you're considering dentistry as a career for the right reasons. Are you a practical sort of person? I mean, do you like working with your hands because manual dexterity is very important in dentistry?'

'Not really, but don't they teach you all that stuff?'

'You receive instructions and training but unless you're a practical person you'll find it difficult. Have you made model boats or aircraft or done any woodwork, or drawing – anything like that?'

'No, I wouldn't know which end of a screwdriver to hold but I'm sure I could soon learn. Plumbers and electricians are practical people but they haven't much brain, have they? I'm sure if they can do practical things, anyone can if they have to.'

'I wouldn't be too sure about that if I were you. Most plumbers and electricians are very skilled in their own fields and you shouldn't denigrate them. And make no mistake about it; dentistry requires a considerable degree of manual ability. Do you realize that most of the time you are working upside down and back to front through a mirror with water spraying everywhere preventing you from getting a clear view of what you're doing? Not to mention having to cope with lips, cheeks and tongues getting in the way.'

Hubert shrugged. 'Sounds difficult when you describe it in that way but it's probably like most things in life – it becomes easy when you've done it a few times.'

After speaking to Hubert for a few minutes I had come to appreciate what Spencer meant when he said he thought he was over-confident; it appeared to me that he had a very arrogant outlook on life and other people, which wasn't at all endearing. I decided to take him into my surgery to prepare for my next patient who was Mr Mellor, coming to have impressions taken for some new dentures.

'Do you make a lot of false teeth? Hubert asked with a look of disdain.

'Yes, quite a lot.'

'Not very glamorous is it – messing about with false teeth?'

'It's an essential part of the job. If you didn't have your own teeth you'd be glad of someone to make you some dentures.'

'But why on earth do people lose all their teeth? It must be because they couldn't be bothered to look after them, so they wouldn't get a lot of sympathy from me.'

174

'People can lose their teeth for many reasons and, in any case, it's not for us to pass judgement. Though from what you've told me so far, I imagine you'd be very happy to take their money for making them dentures.'

'How much do you charge?'

'Depends on the materials – some denture teeth are more expensive than others, and we may adjust the fee according to the degree of difficulty we expect to encounter, but about sixty pounds for a full set.'

'Sixty quid?' spluttered Hubert. 'Crikey, that's not bad for some bits of plastic. I told you dentists can rake it in.'

'It's not as easy as you might think and don't forget that you have to pay a technician for the laboratory work involved.'

'But they aren't professionals, are they? They're just tradesmen so they can't charge that much.'

I didn't like the way Hubert looked down his nose at people just because they weren't doing jobs that he considered to be high-powered. 'There you go again, Hubert, speaking disparagingly without justification. Dental technicians do an important job and most of them are very highly skilled. If you go to dental school you'll have to do some laboratory work as part of your training and you'll soon realize that it's not easy.'

'You mean dental students have to actually make false teeth?'

'I certainly did when I was at university; and crowns and bridges.'

Hubert scoffed. 'I can't see the point in that when you'll be paying a technician to do the work for you after you're qualified.'

'But how can you supervise the technician's work unless you are able to do it yourself?'

Hubert shrugged but didn't answer and I don't think for one moment that I had convinced him of anything. For someone so young and with little experience of life he seemed to have some very strong views.

CHAPTER TWENTY SEVEN

I was quite relieved to reach the end of the morning. Hubert had bombarded me with a whole series of very tiresome questions, most of which were centered on money rather than anything to do with the procedure I was carrying out. He showed very little interest in the actual treatment and didn't appreciate the skill involved. Each time I reached for a piece of equipment he asked how much it cost and how often it needed to be replaced. He wanted to know how much I would be paid for every item of treatment I performed and I am quite sure that when lunchtime arrived he knew far better than I did exactly how much I had earned during the time he had watched me working. I could see that Wendy was not terribly impressed by him and did her best to get on with her work, refusing to allow his presence in the surgery to hinder her. Whenever he asked a money-orientated question she looked at me with an expression that suggested she considered his preoccupation with the financial aspects of dentistry to be inappropriate. When he asked her point blank how much she was paid, she made it quite obvious she thought that he had definitely overstepped the mark.

'That's none of your business,' came her uncharacteristically blunt reply.

As I hung my operating coat on the hook behind my surgery door prior to going for lunch, her exasperation came to the fore. 'Tell me he won't be coming back this afternoon!'

'I'm afraid he will. We're stuck with him for two or three days. Spencer knew what he was doing when he palmed him off onto me. I shan't forgive him in a hurry.'

I returned from lunch just before two o'clock. Wendy was still out, Spencer was taking his customary post-prandial nap and I knew Beryl was going to be late back because she had asked for permission to take time to visit a friend who was unwell. I was surprised, therefore, when I heard voices. I soon realized one of them belonged to Hubert and he was talking to someone in my surgery.

'I really think you ought to go ahead and have all your front teeth crowned,' I heard him say.

'I am thinking about it but I know it will cost an awful lot of money and I don't honestly think I can afford it,' came a female's reply.

'But can you afford not to? Just think what it will do for your appearance – your chances of finding a husband will be greatly enhanced. Surely you don't want to remain a spinster all your life? I don't mean to be unkind but your teeth aren't very attractive at present and you'll find that members of the opposite sex will be far more interested in you if your teeth look good.'

My first reaction was to barge in and put an immediate stop to this improper conversation between Hubert and my patient, Miss Southern, but surprisingly, she didn't seem particularly upset by what he was saying to her and something made me decide to listen a while longer before making my entrance.

'Do you really think it will improve my chances with men?'

'No doubt about it. You could be a very attractive woman if you paid more attention to your appearance. Once you've got your new smile I suggest you let your hair grow longer and dye it blond, and you should wear more make-up. It would also be a good thing if you wore brighter clothes and shorter skirts. As for the expense – look at it this way, you could spend far more on a week's holiday and at the end of the week when it's all over you've nothing to show for it whilst the crowns will be with you all day and every day forever after. Compared with the cost of, for example a new car, it isn't very much at all, is it?'

'I don't know exactly how much it would cost; I haven't discussed it with Mr Derwent but I imagine it would be expensive.'

'Until you ask, you don't know. It might cost a lot less than you think. At least it's worth finding out.'

'I suppose so, Mr Hubert. If I did decide to go ahead would you do the treatment or Mr Derwent?'

'Oh Mr Derwent. You are his patient after all, and I wouldn't want to steal you from him. I'm merely offering you some advice.'

I decided that the time had come for me to intervene.

'Good afternoon, Miss Southern. Please take a seat and I'll be with you very shortly. Hubert, a word please, in the office!'

'What on earth do you think you're doing?' I demanded as soon as I had Hubert on his own.

'I was persuading Miss Southern to have her front teeth crowned. You should be pleased that I'm drumming up business for you. If you crown her six upper and lower front teeth, I should imagine it'll be quite lucrative.'

'You have no business to be talking to patients about their treatment – you're not qualified and to be saying that it will improve her chances with men is absolutely unforgivable.'

'I think it will. She's not a bad looking woman; she could be quite attractive if she smartened herself up and I think crowning her teeth would give her confidence a boost.'

'You also led her to believe that you're a dentist which is totally unacceptable.'

'I didn't tell her I was a dentist – she just assumed.'

'I'm sorry, Hubert, but I can't allow you to take it on yourself to try to influence patients over their choice of treatment. From now on you must not talk to patients unless I or Mr Padginton is present.'

Hubert shrugged in a way that suggested he couldn't see that he had done anything wrong and I went to my surgery to see Miss Southern. I didn't invite Hubert to join me but he followed nevertheless.

'Mr Hubert seems to think it would be a good idea for me to have my front teeth crowned, Mr Derwent. What do you think?'

'It has to be your decision, Miss Southern. It wouldn't be right for me to try to pressurize you. My role is to explain the possible courses of treatment available, give you an estimate of the cost, and point out the advantages and any potential disadvantages.'

'But Mr Hubert said he thought it would improve my chances with the opposite sex. Do you think it would?'

'It isn't for me to speculate on that and he shouldn't have said it to you. By crowning your teeth we can straighten them and make them whiter which I think would improve their appearance but there would be quite a lot of drilling involved, which you might not be prepared to undergo and to have the upper and lowers crowned it would cost £350.'

Miss Southern's face suddenly lit up. 'It is considerably less than a new car – Mr Hubert was right. I've already thought about what he said and now I know that the cost is within my means I see no reason why I shouldn't go ahead with the crowns – that's if you're prepared to do them for me Mr Derwent. Though I suppose I could always get Mr. Hubert to do them, if you aren't willing.'

Hubert gave me a smug grin which I found extremely annoying but I had to admit that his sales patter appeared to have got through to Miss Southern. I was about to tell her that Hubert wasn't a qualified dentist but then I decided against it. 'Of course I would be happy to do the crowns for you if you would like me to.'

A second wave of annoyance swept over me when I heard Hubert whisper 'I'll bet you would,' loudly enough to be sure that I would hear, though hopefully, sufficiently muffled for his utterance to be below Miss Southern's hearing threshold.

For the whole of the time I was treating Miss Southern, Hubert bore a self-satisfied expression and I knew he couldn't wait for her to leave so that he could gloat by way of retaliation because I had told him off.

'You might be a good dentist, Justin, but you need to be more forceful if you want to succeed as a businessman – after all, general practice dentistry is very much a business and dentists can go bust just like any other small business. Do you know that seven dental practices in the United Kingdom went bankrupt last year? I did some research and I was surprised when I discovered that; but it just goes to show. If it hadn't been for my helping you out, you would have missed a golden opportunity to sell some private dentistry. She didn't need much persuading and you can't really say I forced her but you hadn't even tried to sell her some crowns.'

'I see my role as providing necessary dental care to patients – not *selling* dentistry like some door-to-door salesman,' I replied haughtily.

I found his self-assured, superior attitude extremely hard to accept particularly in view of his age and I was exceedingly irritated by the pep talk I was receiving from him but at the same time I could see that he was making a valid point. It was true that, rightly or wrongly, I didn't really look upon dentistry as a business. I did see dentistry as a caring profession and foremost in my mind was that I had a duty to provide what was in the patient's best interests rather than go looking for treatment that would help to swell my bank balance. But I had to admit that on this occasion it appeared that crowning Miss Southern's front teeth was in her best interests – she certainly seemed to think so. By not suggesting the crowns, it could be said that I was failing in my duty to inform her of all the treatment options available to her. I hadn't even considered she might want to have her front teeth crowned but Hubert had, and on reflection, maybe I should have thought about it. But where do you draw the line on this? I couldn't possibly explain all possible treatments to every patient I saw; there simply wasn't enough time.

This conundrum troubled me for a while and at the end of the day when Hubert and Wendy had gone home I spoke to Spencer about it. He adopted the expression I had come to recognize as indicating that he was considering my question with due deference and was about to make a profound statement based on experience. The corners of his mouth turned down and his chin puckered. As he slowly lifted his head, he drew in a deep breath, his brow furrowed and his eyelids fluttered momentarily, then he spoke.

'You can't possibly explain every possible treatment to every patient but it's important to look at the patient as an individual rather than just a set of teeth and you need to make every attempt to assess what treatments might be appropriate for him or her. We should remember that patients can't possibly know all that's available unless we tell them. In the case of Miss Southern; she is a young unmarried woman with front teeth that are somewhat irregular, stained and with fairly big rather unsightly fillings. We ought to recognize that someone like her might be interested in some cosmetic work and I don't think it's the slightest bit unethical to ask if she has ever considered it. It only becomes unethical if we apply undue pressure. Young Hubert is actually quite right when he says that general practice dentistry is a business and unfortunately we do need to keep the bank manager happy, which means we have to show a profit at the end of the year. There's no doubt that this type of work is highly profitable.

'Because Hubert isn't a dentist he is unfettered by the professionalism which may tend to inhibit us and whilst some of the things he said to Miss Southern were a bit out of order you can't deny that he managed to get through to her. He has landed you a nice little job, Justin, and you ought to be grateful to him. He might be young, but he was very quick to spot her weakness and exploit it to his, or on this occasion, your advantage. It seems to me that he probably has a better understanding of women than you.'

CHAPTER TWENTY EIGHT

I decided I would have to take the bull by the horns and ask Harriet to go out with me. I very much wanted to see her again and I couldn't just sit back and hope she might phone me. She had done all the running so far and I couldn't expect her to go on doing it. The last time I saw her I promised I would get in touch with her so why hadn't I done so? I was actually well aware of the reason for my hesitancy – it was Sarah. I didn't feel that I could go out with Harriet many more times without telling Sarah about her. At present I wasn't sure whether it was likely there would ever be anything serious between Harriet and me and I had decided that until I knew, there was no point in saying anything to Sarah. However, I thought that if I were to ask Harriet out on a proper date and let her know how I felt about her, some of the uncertainty I was experiencing at present might be removed. I found uncertainty in life difficult to cope with so it was important that I should try to eliminate it as quickly as possible.

The telephone seemed to go ringing for ages and I was beginning to think there was no-one at home. I was on the point of hanging up when a female voice answered.

'Hello, can I speak to Harriet, please?'

'Who's calling?'

'It's Justin Derwent.' I knew immediately that I was speaking to her mother.

'Oh hello, Justin. How are you?'

'I'm very well, thank you. How are you?'

'Yes we're fine. I must apologize for phoning you the other evening but it was getting late and I was beginning to worry about Harriet. You can understand how I felt, can't you? I didn't know anything about you other than that you're a dentist. Mothers can't help worrying about their daughters, you know.'

'I can understand that. I didn't mind you phoning though I don't think Harriet was altogether happy about it.'

'No, she was furious. She said "whatever will he think? In fact, what were *you* thinking of, mother, to phone him at that time of night? It wasn't as though you even know him." But that's exactly why I phoned, because I didn't know you or anything about you. You could have been married or anything for all I knew.'

I wasn't at all sure what she had in mind when she said 'or anything'.

'I understand why you phoned,' I replied, 'really I do. Is Harriet there? Can I speak to her?'

'Yes she's here; I'll get her for you,' she replied, but made no attempt to do so immediately. 'Have you lived on your own for very long?' she continued.

Before I had time to answer I heard Harriet say indignantly, 'give me the phone, mother.'

There was a minor scuffle at the other end and I had a vision of Harriet wrenching the handset out of her mother's hand.

'Hello, Justin, I'm really sorry about that; my mother's terrible. She has the knack of being able to squeeze out someone's entire life history within ten minutes of meeting them. How are you?'

'I'm fine thank you, Harriet. Are you well?'

'Yes, I'm all right. I'm not looking forward to the sex education lesson I'm due to give tomorrow but apart from that.'

'Oh, poor you. I certainly don't envy you having to do that but I'm sure you'll be brilliant.'

'I very much doubt it. I don't think I'm going to be able to go on talking around the subject much longer before one of the little horrors demands that I get down to the nitty-gritty. I'm convinced they're just hell-bent on embarrassing me and are taking great delight in watching me squirm. It's a complete waste of time really because it's quite obvious there isn't anything I could teach them they don't already know. I shall just be glad when it's all over.'

'Would it cheer you up if I offered to take you out to dinner?'

'It certainly would, Justin. That would be really lovely, thank you, when did you have in mind?'

'What about this evening? I know it's short notice but I would love to see you if you aren't doing anything else.'

'This evening? Oh, err, well, yes, I haven't any other plans. Will you give me time to get ready?'

'I'll pick you up in half-an-hour if that's all right.'

'Could you possibly give me a little bit longer, please?'

'Of course, how long do you need?'

'Can we say an hour?' she replied almost beseechingly.

'An hour it is then.'

Exactly sixty minutes later I rang Harriet's doorbell and her mother opened the door.

She was an attractive lady in her forties with short fair hair and a face which broke into a smile very easily revealing a set of nice white teeth. She was smartly dressed and shorter than Harriet but probably somewhat heavier.

'Hello Justin, I'm very pleased to meet you, do come in, Harriet won't be very long – I think she's nearly ready. You certainly threw her into a spin when you said you'd give her an hour to get ready. It takes her more than an hour to wash and dry her hair, and then she's got to have a bath and get dressed.'

I heard Harriet call, 'I'm coming.' She might have got herself ready in a hurry but it certainly didn't show – she looked amazing as she walked down the stairs. Her freshly-shampooed, auburn hair cascaded over her pale unblemished skin and her eyes looked bluer and clearer than ever. My gaze locked on to hers and we both held it for several seconds until the merest flush of embarrassment coloured her cheeks and she looked away. At that moment, for some inexplicable reason I suddenly had the feeling that fate had decreed that our futures would somehow become intertwined.

'You look absolutely lovely,' I said before I could think what I was saying – not that there was anything particularly wrong in saying that but it did cause Harriet a second and slightly more pronounced flush of embarrassment probably because of her mother's presence.

'I promise we won't be late, Mrs Brooks, I'm working tomorrow and I know Harriet has a difficult day ahead of her.' Harriet's expression told me that she had a sinking feeling in her stomach just thinking about it.

'As long as I know,' said Harriet's mother, 'and please call me Eileen – Mrs Brooks sounds like someone ancient. Anyway, have a nice time. Where are you planning on going?'

'Mother!' exclaimed Harriet showing obvious disapproval.

'It's just in case I need to contact you.'

'What possible reason could you have for needing to contact me that couldn't wait for me to get home? I'm going out for the evening not going away for a month.'

'I'm sorry about that, Justin; my mother can be quite overbearing at times,' explained Harriet apologetically as soon as we were in my car and on our way.

'That's all right; you don't need to apologize for her. At least she cares.'

'A bit too much at times.'

'Why do you say that?' I asked, though I'd more or less already got the picture.

'She tends to be over-protective and isn't happy unless she knows exactly where I am and what I'm doing. When I wanted to go to university she nearly went mad when I said I was considering London or Edinburgh. In the end she grudgingly agreed to let me go to Southampton because it's the nearest and it wouldn't be too difficult for me to get home from there.'

'At least she didn't stop you going altogether.'

'She probably would have done if she could but I mustn't be too hard on her – she means well, it's just a bit stifling at times.'

'Yes I can see that but you're happy at Southampton, aren't you?'

'The university's all right but I hate the city of Southampton. I'm a country girl really – I love to be surrounded by open space and to see sheep and cows in the fields. I couldn't live in a city, I would go mad. How about you?'

'I'd lived in a city all my life until I came to Luccombury. I like to think I could probably settle anywhere but it's nice to live in the country.'

I took Harriet to a little restaurant I had visited once before. It was very cosy and atmospheric without being too ostentatious and it served excellent food. We had a most enjoyable meal and shared a bottle of wine though I got the impression that Harriet wasn't used to drinking very much. We chatted easily and comfortably throughout the evening about all sorts of things but time was getting on and I was aware that soon we would have finished our coffee and it would be time to head back home. Before we left I was hoping to bring the conversation round to something a little closer to my heart. I reached across the table and took hold of her hand and experienced a warm tinge of encouragement when I felt her respond, and her smile told me that she didn't object to the contact.

'I really like you, Harriet,' I began clumsily and for a moment I didn't have a clue what to say next. I think Harriet was about to reply but held back because she sensed I was going to say something else. After what seemed like an interminable hesitation I continued with 'I would very much like to see you again, if you would like to.'

'I like you too, Justin. There's just one thing I find very worrying – a girl with sleek, blond hair you've been seeing recently, perhaps you're still seeing her.'

'Ah, you mean Sarah. I've been out with her a few times but I can honestly say that it was never serious and it's definitely over now.'

'You went out with her on Saturday evening – the day after you took me for a drink which isn't that long ago so when did you finish with her?'

'I told her it was over between us on Saturday.' I felt my conscience prick me as I said it but I couldn't let Harriet think I was still seeing Sarah. I hoped my expression and body language weren't indicating that I wasn't telling the truth and I was very aware that Harriet, being a student of psychology would be very quick to see through my dishonesty. 'But how did you know I went out with her on Saturday?'

'My mother saw you. She wasn't sure it was you because she didn't know you but she thought she recognized your car – it seems she was right. She was horrible about it. She said "he was with this woman with lovely sleek blond hair, not a single hair out of place, she looked very glamorous. You won't stand a chance against her".'

I was beginning to think it was a very small world around Luccombury and that it was virtually impossible to do anything without someone observing your actions. However, I was heartened to hear that Harriet and her mother had given consideration to Harriet's 'chances' with me. Maybe she was genuinely interested in me after all. 'It sounds as though your mother doesn't approve of me very much.' I sighed with a tinge of sadness in my voice.

'It's not that; she'd be the same with anyone. I took a boy from university back home last week and she gave him the third degree. She's simply reserving judgement until she knows more about you though she is concerned, as I am, that there might be someone else in your life. When I first mentioned you to her she was sure you would be married. When I told her you lived alone she then decided you must be divorced. You're not, are you?'

'No, I'm not. I can assure you I've never been married.' I looked for a flicker of relief on Harriet's face but I can't, in all honesty say I detected one. I know I felt a strong pang of jealousy when I thought of her with someone who might be even loosely described as her boyfriend. 'Is it serious between you and the boy you took home last week?' I queried.

'No he's just a friend.' Harriet brushed aside the inference that she might have someone else in her life and seemed more interested in establishing the state of my relationship with Sarah. 'And you say that it's definitely over between you and Sarah?'

As I strived to sound convincing I was aware of Harriet's beautiful eyes boring into me, watching for the slightest twitch, flinch or faltering and I felt as if I was wired up to a lie detector. 'It's definitely over.' I was able to say with considerable conviction because, although I hadn't actually told Sarah yet, I knew in my own mind that I wanted it to be over so that I would be free to see more of Harriet. I hoped she would want to see more of me though she had to be convinced that I was free of encumbrances.

The next step now for me was to face Sarah and break the news to her.

CHAPTER TWENTY NINE

As I started to climb the stairs at the practice next morning I heard the unmistakeable sound of a high-speed dental drill. My first thought was that Spencer must have started work early but then I remembered that his surgery was now downstairs and this was coming from upstairs – coming from my surgery, so what could it be?

The door was open and I was greeted by the sight of Hubert, dental drill in hand, operating on a set of plastic teeth which he had placed on the bracket table. He had made no attempt to catch the water spray which was shooting out from the head of the drill shrouding him in a wet mist and creating large pools of water on the surgery floor all around the chair. He was so engrossed in what he was doing he didn't see me arrive and I deliberately startled him.

'Have you any idea how much those hand pieces cost?' I demanded sternly.

'Oh, hello, Justin, I didn't see you. I'm just having a go at drilling a tooth. I don't think I'm making a bad job of it what do you think?' He handed the plastic model to me.

'What exactly do you think you're doing? There's more to it than just drilling holes, you know. The cavity has to be prepared in a particular way depending on where the decay is situated and how you intend to restore the tooth.'

'I suppose there is a bit more to it than just drilling a hole but there can't be much more. It looks simple enough to me. I was wondering if you'd let me have a go on a patient this morning.'

'Don't be ridiculous, Hubert, you know I can't let you do that. You aren't qualified.'

'I don't see why not. You had to start somewhere. You weren't qualified when you treated your first patient so what's the difference?'

'The difference is that I had undergone several months of practical instructions on a phantom head under the guidance of qualified instructors who had to be satisfied that I was competent before I was let loose on the public. There is no way I'm going to allow you to treat a patient – you are here to watch only. Is that clear?'

'I suppose so but it gets a bit boring just watching – I want to get in on the action.'

'Well if you want to get in on the action you can start by mopping up all that water from the floor. You'd better get on with it before Wendy arrives or she'll be furious with you.'

'All right, I'll clean it up,' he said resignedly then his face lit up again as another idea came to him. 'Surely I could act as dental nurse. I've watched what Wendy does and I'm sure I could suck out saliva and mix filling materials. I could do that, couldn't I? It would be more interesting than just watching.'

I wasn't at all keen but I knew he would keep on until I agreed so reluctantly I said 'I'm doing a root filling first thing this morning and I shall need Wendy to help me with that but then, providing she agrees, you can take over from her and help me later on.'

'Thanks, Justin, that's great. I won't let you down, just as long as you promise not to play footsy with me under the chair whilst we're working,' he replied cheekily.

'You can most definitely rest assured on that, Hubert,' I replied frostily.

I don't think Wendy thought it was a particularly good idea when I told her that she was going to be replaced for part of the morning but because she had a considerable amount of paperwork to catch up on she was thankful for the opportunity to work in the office though I told her to listen carefully and come straight to the surgery if I called her.

Although I had some reservations about letting Hubert assist me I tried to convince myself that he couldn't really do any harm and I resolved to stop him immediately if he started to step out of line. What I had overlooked, however, was that the first patient we would be treating after he assumed his new role was a certain Claudia Verity. Claudia was in her early twenties and was guaranteed to turn the head of any red-blooded male the right side of ninety. In fact he didn't really need to be all that red-blooded to be lured by her. Wendy escorted her from the waiting room by way of her final duty before handing over the role of dental nurse for the rest of the morning to Hubert and she raised her eyes at me in disapproval of Claudia's attire.

As soon as Claudia wiggled into my surgery, Hubert's jaw dropped to his waist and I'm sure he couldn't believe what he was witnessing. I was close behind him at that moment and I said to him quietly, 'I'd close your mouth if I were you, Hubert, you might swallow a fly,' though in the circumstances I wasn't altogether surprised at his reaction.

Claudia was extremely buxom with long, straight, bleached-blond hair and was wearing high heels and a leather skirt which was at least twelve inches above her knees. Her pink, silk blouse had a daringly plunging neckline and the tiny pearl buttons looked as if they would at any moment, fail in their struggle to maintain her decency. Hubert couldn't take his eyes off her and appeared to be completely mesmerised. 'Would you like to come and take a seat, Claudia,' he announced suddenly before I had a chance to make the same offer though I would have addressed her as 'Miss Verity.'

Claudia was not the most talkative of girls, at least that had been my experience of her so far, and she sat in the dental chair without saying a word. Most of her concentration was taken up with pulling on the hem of her skirt in a vain attempt to cover up the vast area of exposed thigh which was currently dominating Hubert's attention. 'What are we doing today?' he asked of me as he strained to read the patient's notes I was holding in my hand.

'We're fitting a crown on an upper premolar,' I responded.

For the first time since Claudia arrived, Hubert looked at her face. 'Today we're going fit a crown to your upper premolar,' he announced.

'Thank you, Hubert.' I interjected. 'Will you put a bib on Miss Verity, please?'

I was sure I heard Hubert say 'shame' but I couldn't swear to it and I don't think Claudia heard him because there was no reaction from her.

'The tooth has already been prepared for the crown,' I explained, 'so there won't be much drilling but I do need to take off the temporary crown and it might be a bit sensitive. Would you prefer to have an injection?' Naturally I was speaking to Claudia but Hubert interjected.

'Prefer it over what?' he demanded.

'Over not having one,' I expounded. 'It might be a bit sensitive so some people will want an injection; other people might decide that as the pain is only slight they'll manage without an injection. It's a matter of personal preference.'

'But they won't know till they've tried it, will they? I thought you were going to offer some innovative, new, alternative method of pain control,' grinned Hubert.

'I'm afraid not – it's an injection or nothing. Many people have an idea whether their teeth are sensitive or not and whether or not they are prepared to suffer some slight discomfort. If they don't have any thoughts on the subject then I decide for them and I always go for the injection.' I turned to Claudia, 'would you like me to give you an injection before we start?'

'I don't want it to hurt,' said Claudia screwing up her face.

'Very well then – an injection it is. Hubert, will you pass me the topical anaesthetic paste, please. That's to deaden the gum before I inject,' I explained to him.

'I know, I know,' he replied indignantly, 'I've seen you use it before.' Then he turned to Claudia and without hesitation he announced, 'he's just going to rub something on so you don't feel the prick when it goes in.' His words were accompanied by a wildly exaggerated demonstration of giving an injection which was more like a vet injecting a horse than any procedure a dentist would ever carry out.

'Hubert, a word please, now, in the office.'

He followed me out of the surgery shrugging his shoulders and bearing a scornful expression.

'I can't believe that you could be so stupid as to say something like that. Many patients would understandably be very offended in fact, they would be fully justified in making a formal complaint but the complaint will be against me not you because you are only here as an observer. I'm the one who will be held responsible.'

'I didn't say anything wrong,' protested Hubert.

'You don't think so? Well if you can't see it then the only safe way from now on is for you to keep your mouth shut. I have no desire to be hauled up before the GDC or appear on the front page of the *News of the World* because of your stupidity. Now let's get back to work and don't let me hear you say another word in front of a patient.'

I was relieved that Claudia appeared to be completely oblivious to the possible implications of Hubert's words and displayed no reaction whatsoever. As soon as I had administered the injection I said to Claudia 'Would you like to rinse out your mouth, Miss Verity.' I sensed that Hubert was about to say something but my withering look reminded him that he had to remain silent.

The injection took effect quickly and I was able to able to remove the temporary crown and clean up the prepared tooth without Claudia feeling any pain. The finished crown matched the colour of her other teeth extremely well and it also fitted perfectly but as was sometimes the case, it was a little bit too high on the bite and met the lower teeth prematurely when she closed her teeth together. It was a fairly common problem and easily rectified; all that was needed was to identify the high spot, grind a little bit off, and polish it smooth.

Each time I tried in the crown to see if I had removed enough material Claudia reached for the glass of mouthwash and insisted on rinsing and spitting several times in order to clear her mouth of the small amount of debris that was created by the grinding. I didn't mind this though it did tend to make the job take longer. Hubert on the other hand was positively enjoying it because all her activity was gradually dislodging her bib and providing him with an enjoyable diversion. Had Wendy been assisting me she would have repositioned the bib immediately but Hubert made no attempt to do this probably because he found the view without the bib far more interesting. I was too intent on adjusting the crown to notice that the bib was no longer protecting Claudia's silk blouse from possible contamination from the procedure.

Having established that I had ground enough off the biting surface, all that remained was to re-polish the crown before cementing it in place. The first stage of the polishing was achieved by means of a special rubber wheel and then, a small felt mop charged with a suitable compound completed the process by achieving a high gloss. One of the problems encountered with a small crown is that it can be very difficult to keep a firm grip on it during the polishing because there isn't much to hold on to and the rapidly revolving instruments can easily dislodge it from your fingers and that's exactly what happened on this occasion.

Sometimes the crown can fly some considerable distance through the air and many dental restorations have been lost forever in this way. It's amazing how they manage to disappear down cracks between the floorboards, down the sink, behind a radiator or even out of an open window. On this occasion the crown didn't fly too far but the consequences were no less devastating. It left my fingers and shot along a straight trajectory landing fairly and squarely in the middle of Claudia's sunburnt chest before sliding tantalisingly slowly down her ample cleavage where it finally disappeared from view.

Hubert had followed its progress like a hawk and quick as a flash he thrust his hand along the same pathway with total disregard for propriety, dignity or the integrity of her pearl buttons, two of which were torn off, ripping open her blouse to reveal an alluring, pink lacy undergarment.

Up to that moment, Claudia's movements had been fairly sluggish but suddenly she sprang into action. She shrieked and leapt up out of the chair dragging Hubert with her. Her left hand seized his wrist and dragged his sinful fingers from the forbidden territory whilst her right hand delivered a crashing blow to his cheek. It appeared that Hubert had located the crown and had it in his grasp until Claudia's counterattack caused him to drop it onto the floor. I was horrified at Hubert's thoughtless behaviour, but at the same time I found it very difficult to refrain from laughing because the whole incident was highly comical, though I'm quite sure Claudia didn't think so, and judging by the way Hubert was rubbing his cheek and exercising his jaw, I would say that he wasn't amused either.

'Just look what you've done to my blouse,' were Claudia's first words. 'You'll pay for this; I want a new blouse.'

I stepped in rapidly to try to diffuse the situation. 'I'm so sorry about your blouse, Miss Verity; please accept my sincere apologies for my assistant's behaviour; he was quite out of order.'

'I want a new blouse,' she insisted, 'he's ruined this one.'

'It only needs the buttons sewing back on,' chimed in Hubert whose cheek was getting redder by the minute.

'Hubert, will you please leave this to me? Go into the office and get Wendy to come in and assist me. You've done enough damage for one day!'

I thought Hubert was about to persist with his protest but he didn't – he decided to go quietly though he didn't need to summon Wendy; she had heard the commotion and was already on her way. She arrived as I was continuing to try and calm down Claudia and I saw a look of shock when she saw that Claudia's blouse was revealing even more than when she had first arrived. 'Let me cover you with a new bib,' she said soothingly.

'I'm so sorry about your blouse, Miss Verity, of course we'll buy you a new one. Do you know how much it will cost to replace it?'

'I only bought it yesterday; it cost me £4.'

'Then will you be happy if I deduct £4 from your dental bill?'

'I suppose so,' she replied grumpily.

'Thank you for being so understanding. I'll fit your crown and then I'll get Wendy to make you a cup of tea before you go. Would you like that?'

'Yes thank you,' she responded looking marginally happier, then her countenance changed. 'He won't be coming back, will he?' she asked with alarm in her voice.

'No, I'll get Wendy to assist me.'

'Thank heaven for that.'

After I'd finished with Claudia I went into the office where Hubert was sitting looking grumpily out of the window.

'That was a bloody stupid thing to do, Hubert. Didn't you think what you were doing and consider the consequences of your actions?'

'I was just intent on retrieving the crown – I didn't mean any harm.'

'Maybe you didn't but if you go around thrusting your hand down women's blouses you're going to have one hell of a time proving your innocence, in fact you'll be lucky not to get yourself locked up. You were damned lucky to get away with it today. I said earlier that you needed to think before you speak, you obviously need to think before you act as well. Consider yourself very fortunate that I'm not asking you to pay for her new blouse.'

'She doesn't need a new blouse,' Hubert insisted. 'If she sews the buttons back on it'll be fine. I wouldn't have agreed to buy her a new one.'

'In a situation like this it's vital that you do whatever is necessary to smooth things over. You assaulted her, there's no other way of putting it and she could report you to the police which is the last thing you want so you don't start quibbling with her. If buying her a new blouse will placate her then that's what you have to do.'

Hubert grunted and I wasn't sure whether my message had got through to him or not. After looking thoughtful for a few moments he spoke.

'I was only trying to be helpful by retrieving the crown. I'll be more careful next time,' he promised. 'I think the problem is that I don't feel I'm sufficiently involved in the treatment and I want to take a more active role. If you let me do that instead of just watching or assisting I'd probably be better because my mind would be more focussed on the actual job. I see you've got someone coming in for an extraction in a minute, will you let me take the tooth out?'

Words failed me. What could you possibly say to someone like Hubert? I fully understood now why Spencer didn't want to have anything to do with him but even he could not have foreseen the sort of problems an overconfident, unthinking seventeen year old could create in such a short time. My patience with him had run out.

'Of course I won't let you take out a tooth, Hubert. I'm amazed after all that's happened that you've the nerve to ask. I'm sorry but I'm not prepared to have you in my surgery any longer – I simply can't afford to risk you causing any more trouble.'

CHAPTER THIRTY

I felt almost sick to my stomach but I knew I had to do it. I hated hurting people particularly when they didn't really deserve to be hurt and Sarah hadn't done anything wrong but sadly I just felt that she was not the one for me. I wanted to see more of Harriet and I knew it wasn't fair on either of them if I kept on seeing them both and there was also a very real danger that I might upset them both with disastrous results. I couldn't afford to delay any longer and I simply had to tell Sarah that I didn't think we had a future together but I wasn't looking forward to breaking the news to her and I wasn't at all sure how she would take it.

I kept telling myself that I was being ridiculous. Sarah and I had only been out together a few times so you couldn't in all honesty say it was a serious relationship. Until you had been out with someone a number of times it was impossible to know whether or not you were suited to each other and unless you accepted that you would remain with the first girl you ever met for the rest of your life, there were bound to be break-ups and it was kinder to everyone if, once you knew your true feelings, you acted on them sooner rather than later. Richard Darcy didn't seem to have any trouble breaking up with women so why was I finding it so difficult?

I had phoned Sarah and arranged to see her. When I spoke to her, somehow I got the feeling she didn't seem quite as pleased to hear from me as usual, as if there was something on her mind that was troubling her, though I wondered if it was just my imagination fuelled by my own feelings of guilt, fear and uncertainty as to how I would go about telling her. However, she agreed to meet me readily enough and I went to pick her up at her home.

When she greeted me with a simple 'Hello, Justin,' and a quick peck on the cheek, I knew that she was feeling a bit cool towards me for some reason. It was almost as if she knew why I had asked to see her though realistically I couldn't see how that could be possible unless she was telepathic.

I didn't know whether to come straight out with it as soon as we were in my car together or whether I should at least buy her a drink first. I decided that I would probably make a better job of it if I had a stiff drink myself before broaching the subject so I tried my best to keep our conversation flowing freely but inconsequentially until we reached a suitable public house. As it turned out we went to the pub where I had taken Harriet. I didn't plan it that way but as I was more concerned with what I was going to say to Sarah than on my driving, it was almost as if my car had found its own way there. I ordered some drinks and made for a table in a corner so that we could talk without anyone else overhearing.

Having drunk half of my pint of bitter in record time I decided that it was now or never. 'Th…There's something I have to say to you, Sarah,' I don't think you'll be very happy when I tell you but I'm afraid it has to be said.'

'I've a good idea what it is,' she replied quickly before I had to time to elaborate.

'Have you? What do you mean?'

'I think I know what you are about to say.'

'Do you? I don't see how you can.'

'I have my sources of information – there's quite an efficient grapevine around here and I maintain close contact with many of the grapes.'

'I see,' I responded in amazement. I had already said to Harriet that I thought it was a small world around Luccombury– it seemed it wasn't just small; it was miniscule. But how did Sarah know? Could she have seen me out with Harriet or was it someone else who saw me? If it was someone else, it had to be someone who knew Sarah and me, which narrowed the field considerably. I couldn't really think of anyone – I was totally baffled.

'I'm really sorry, Sarah, I hate to do this to you but I've thought about it very carefully before arriving at my decision,' I continued, hoping that she would see that I was genuinely remorseful about the situation.

'It's just one of those things. You can't help the way you feel but I can't deny that I'm very, very disappointed – gutted in fact.'

'But how did you know? You say that there's a very good grapevine around here but I can't think of anyone who would be in a position to be able to tell you.'

I was very surprised that Sarah appeared to be taking it so remarkably well – she seemed to be quite philosophical about it and I began to feel greatly relieved. I had half expected her to fly into a temper, slap my face and storm out. I knew from past experience she could be volatile and I really thought that finding out that I had another girlfriend would have been enough to light her fuse.

'Well,' explained Sarah, 'it was Richard Darcy who spread the message. You told him, and he was discussing it with his friend John in a pub somewhere and they were overheard by a girl I used to work with called Nicola, who I go out with occasionally. She knows Richard Darcy because he dated her some time ago. He didn't see her sitting at the next table in the pub or if he did, he didn't recognize her but I suppose he's dated so many women he can't possibly remember them all.'

'Yes there can't be many around here he hasn't been out with?'

'Well you know my views on Richard Darcy. Anyway he was talking to John about you and me. Nicola doesn't like Richard after the way he treated her and she didn't think it was right that he should be discussing us. After all, it's none of his business.'

As Sarah was speaking, my mind was working overtime trying to think how Richard could possibly have known about Harriet. I felt sure that the last time I spoke to him about her was when I told him that she had come to see me as a patient, that I liked the look of her and he told me I was stupid for not asking her out there and then. I felt pretty sure I hadn't spoken to him since, so he wouldn't have known that I had actually been out with her and that I was planning on finishing with Sarah. Something didn't quite make sense here.

'What exactly did Nicola hear Richard Darcy say?' I enquired with intrigue.

'That nobody in his right mind would even consider jumping out of an aircraft and that it was a ridiculous idea. He said that although you hadn't said definitely you weren't prepared to do it you'd made it clear that the prospect terrified you and he felt sure you had no intention of going through with it. He then went on to say that he thought I must be mad to want to do it and that he had advised you to dump me before I dreamed up any more stupid ventures which could finish up doing you serious harm.'

'Ah, I see,' I spluttered.

'So you can see why I'm so disappointed because you know how badly I wanted us to do the parachute jump together,' sighed Sarah. 'Is what Richard said correct – are you really not prepared to do it with me?'

I was lost for words for some moments. I now realized that Sarah and I had been talking at cross purposes and that she had jumped to the wrong conclusion about what it was I trying to say to her. It wasn't going to be easy after all.

'I don't really see myself jumping out of an aircraft, if I'm honest – I'm sorry to disappoint you, Sarah.' I paused waiting for divine inspiration as to how I should proceed from here and the earlier sense of relief was suddenly replaced by a new and far more profound feeling of apprehension. I took another long swig of beer and noticed that my hand was shaking as I lifted the glass.

'Oh well,' she sighed, 'it was just a dream that may never come to fruition now but never mind; at least you haven't taken Richard's advice and decided to dump me.'

I took hold of her hand and desperately tried to string the right words together. In spite of the fact that I kept gulping mouthfuls of liquid my tongue felt as dry as dust. 'Sarah, I'm very fond of you,' I spluttered, 'really fond of you but I just feel there is something missing in our relationship. I don't know why or what it is but there's something lacking.'

Sarah looked completely puzzled as if my words weren't really making sense to her. She frowned and stared down at the table. 'It's early days, Justin. We hardly know each other yet but we get on well together and we seem to enjoy each other's company. I'm sure we just need to give it more time. I certainly think we should at least try for a bit longer before making any major decisions.'

'I suppose it's because I've only ever been out with one or two girls and I feel that I want to go out with other people before tying myself down to one particular person. I don't feel ready to embark upon a serious relationship at the moment.'

'All men say that even if they've been out with hundreds of different girls. They never think they're ready to settle down,' Sarah replied scornfully.

'I'd like us to remain friends, Sarah, but I don't really want any more than that. I'm truly sorry but that's the way I feel.'

'You've met someone else, haven't you?' Sarah hissed, a hint of venom beginning to creep into her voice.

I wanted to avoid a bitter confrontation if at all possible and I could see that to have any hope of succeeding I would need to tread very carefully. 'No, there isn't anyone else, as I said; I just don't want to be tied down at the moment but I don't want to lose you as a friend.'

'Well, we haven't actually made any sort of commitment to each other,' Sarah responded almost disdainfully, 'we've only been out together a few times, so we're both free to come and go as we like. If that's what you want.'

'I suppose that is what I want but please don't be upset, Sarah; I really don't want to hurt you but I can't help the way I feel.'

'Of course I'm upset, Justin, but at least I know where I stand. I think you'd better take me home now.'

We spoke very little during the journey home. My mind was working overtime and I felt there was more I wanted to say but I knew that it had all been said; I would just be repeating myself. I was thankful when we arrived at Sarah's house because the silence was now quite claustrophobic. I tried desperately, but was unable to think of anything to say that might ease the tension between us which was becoming almost overwhelming.

I brought the car to a standstill outside her house. 'Good night, Sarah,' I said as amicably as I could. She didn't answer but jumped out with a defiant flourish and slammed the door so hard the car rocked violently for some seconds.

CHAPTER THIRTY ONE

I felt somewhat numb after my evening with Sarah. I hated telling her I wanted to end our relationship and there was no doubt that I had upset her. I also felt guilty about the fact that I hadn't been entirely honest with her and that I told her I hadn't met anyone else, which wasn't true. At least I wouldn't be lying to Harriet any longer if I said to her that I had finished with Sarah, though if Harriet knew the whole truth, she might feel that the termination of the relationship wasn't quite as complete as it might have been. All these thoughts were running through my mind and I felt completely unsettled. I almost wanted to phone Sarah and apologize again for upsetting her but I realized that to do so would be completely stupid. I had said what had to be said, more or less; now the best course of action was to wait for the dust to settle.

I thought I might phone Harriet and invite her out. I wanted to see her but I somehow felt that the evening with Sarah was still too fresh in my thoughts and I had to remember that I had told Harriet I had finished with Sarah some days ago. Perhaps it would be advisable to wait a little while before contacting her. I don't really know why I arrived at that conclusion – it seemed a bit illogical but I suppose I felt the need to allow my mind to calm down because at the moment, it was in turmoil.

I telephoned Tom Cox to see if he wanted to go to an exhibition of photography which was being organized by a local camera club. There was no answer and I eventually remembered that the last time I saw him he told me he was planning on going sailing as soon as the weather improved. The weather had been good for the last three days and, according to the forecast, was set fair for some time to come so I assumed that's where he was. I almost resigned myself to an evening at home but then I decided to go to the exhibition alone – I felt sure it would be interesting and it wasn't very far to drive.

The journey to the exhibition took me quite near to where Sarah lived and I wondered how she felt today. I hoped she wasn't too unhappy and the more I thought about it the more convinced I became that she would quickly move on with her life; I felt sure she was that sort of person. She had quite a sharp temper and I had felt the full force of it once or twice but I was pretty certain her outbursts were short lived.

My mind seemed to be working overtime and I don't suppose I was concentrating terribly hard on my driving. It was early evening, the road was dry, visibility was good and there weren't many other cars on the road. Suddenly, my attention was arrested by an orange object which seemed to materialize from nowhere and rapidly zoom towards me like a missile. There was a sickening crunch as metal panels disintegrated and glass smashed. I lurched forward banging my head against the windscreen though miraculously I suffered no serious harm though the same could not be said about my car and my first observation now that I was stationary was that my nearside front wheel was sitting on the passenger seat.

I felt slightly dizzy but I think it was due to shock more than the bang on my head and for some moments I sat in complete disbelief amongst the tangled wreck that, until a few seconds ago had been my pride and joy.

'Are you all right?' were the first words I heard when I finally extricated myself from behind the steering wheel. 'I'm really sorry, I don't know what happened; I just didn't see you.'

A very pale elderly gentleman was tottering towards me looking very shaken and upset but apparently uninjured. His car was in a fairly sorry state as well; with steam issuing from the punctured radiator though the damage appeared not to be as extensive as that sustained by my little sports car. 'Are you all right?' he repeated.

'Yes, I think so. Are you hurt?'

'No, I'm not hurt,' he confirmed. 'I really am terribly sorry; I don't know this road and I thought I had right of way and that the main road went off to the right but I see now that you were on the main road.'

I too was sorry that my car was so badly damaged and my first reaction was that he had been driving carelessly but there was no point in getting annoyed. He had made a mistake, was genuinely sorry and had already done what all insurance companies say you should never do – he had virtually admitted liability. I saw that there were three women still sitting in his car and none of them was making any effort to get out. 'Are your passengers all right?' I asked with some concern.

'Yes I think so. They're a bit shaken just as I am but they aren't hurt. Do you think we could push my car off the main road onto the side road? I don't think we can move yours because the front wheel is off but if we move mine there'll be less of an obstruction to other traffic.'

Together we pushed his car out of the way and then we exchanged names and addresses and insurance details. His three passengers remained in his car throughout without saying a word to each other; each one sat looking straight ahead as if in some sort of stupor.

'Are you a member of the AA?' I asked the other driver.

'No,' he replied. 'I shall phone my brother who is a motor engineer and ask him who I should get in touch with. We're on holiday staying in a guest house quite near to here so I think I'll take the ladies back and phone from there. My car should be all right where it is until someone comes to tow it away.'

'I'm sorry you've had your holiday spoilt.'

'These things happen. It was my fault anyway but it will all get sorted out – at least no one is hurt. What will you do about your car?'

'I'll phone the AA, I believe there's a phone kiosk a bit further down the road.'

'So will you be all right if I take the ladies back to the guest house?'

'Yes, I'll be fine. You go.'

'I'm truly sorry about your car, Mr Derwent. I hope you can get it sorted out.'

We shook hands and as he ushered the three ladies out of his car I looked again at the damage to mine. It was bad and I realized that if I had been carrying a passenger they would probably have been badly hurt. Fortunately for me, the nearside front wing had taken the brunt of the impact and my side of the car was relatively unscathed but the damage was nevertheless quite severe and I doubted if economic repair would be possible. In other words my precious little car was probably a write-off.

The AA said they would send out a recovery vehicle as soon as possible but it could be an hour before it arrived. The information didn't seem to sink in very well as my mind was in an even greater state of confusion now than it had been when I was thinking about Sarah and Harriet. However, it did suddenly occur to me that after the AA had picked up my car, I would be stranded, with no means of getting home. I knew that Sarah lived only a short distance away and I was strongly tempted to go to her house and ask her to give me a lift but I really didn't want to do this after last night. I realized that if I did so there would be one of two possible outcomes. Either she would still be annoyed with me and refuse to help or, more likely, she would be only too willing to come to my rescue, which would have the effect of negating last night's conversation and put us back to where we were previously. I would need to be very hard indeed to take advantage of her kindness then tell her that nothing had changed and that I still wanted to end our relationship. I really didn't know what to do, then entirely on impulse; I walked back to the telephone kiosk and rang Harriet. I was relieved when she and not her mother answered.

'I'm sorry to bother you, Harriet, but I've been involved in a car accident. My car's badly damaged and is going to be towed away by the AA so I will need a lift home. I don't like to ask but is there any chance you could come and pick me up – I really would be most grateful.'

'Oh, Justin, how terrible, are you all right?'

'Yes I'm not hurt.'

'Thank goodness for that. So where are you?'

'On the road between Luccombury and Sonnington, just before you get to the Horse and Hounds public house. Do you know it?'

'Yes I know the road; there are some sharp bends.'

'That's right. It was on one the bends that the crash happened.'

'Sarah lives near there, doesn't she? '

'Yes she does but I don't want to ask her for help now that I've finished with her. Anyway how do you know she lives near here?'

Harriet paused before answering. 'You must have told me.'

'I don't remember telling you, but it doesn't matter. As I said, I don't really want to make contact with her. Can you help me?'

'Of course I will, Justin; I'm on my way. I'll be with you very shortly.'

'That's really kind of you, Harriet; I'm very grateful and please drive carefully.'

'You're a good one to talk having just smashed up your car,' she chuckled. 'See you soon.'

I walked slowly back to my car from the telephone kiosk thinking it was a bit cheeky of me ask Harriet to come and fetch me. We didn't know each other all that well and she might have had other plans for the evening. I then began to wonder again how she knew where Sarah lived. The more I thought about it the more certain I felt that I hadn't told her.

I was expecting her to arrive in her mother's Ford Cortina so it wasn't surprising that I didn't realize it was her when she pulled up alongside me in a little grey Morris 1000.

'Meet Ellie May,' were her opening words to me through the open passenger window. She was smiling until she saw my green sports car and her expression changed to one of horror. 'Oh my God, just look at your car. You were very lucky to escape from that unscathed. Are you sure you aren't hurt?'

'I'm fine. Thank you so much for coming, Harriet, I really do appreciate it. I hope you didn't have other plans this evening.'

'Nothing that couldn't be changed,' she replied.

'So you did have other plans. I'm so sorry I dragged you away; you should have said if it wasn't convenient. What were you intending to do?'

'I had some friends turn up and we were going out. When you phoned I just said I was sorry but I had to go somewhere and I left.'

She sensed that I was feeling guilty about calling her away from her friends and quickly dispelled my concern. 'I was so pleased to hear from you, Justin, and pleased you asked me and not Sarah to help you. I honestly didn't mind coming to fetch you.'

'I can't begin to tell you how grateful I am. I hope the AA won't be long now.'

'We can sit in Ellie May and wait if you like,' she suggested.

'Is she yours?'

'Yes, my uncle got her for me, he's a motor engineer. Don't you think she's lovely?'

'She certainly is. Why do you call her Ellie May?'

'Her registration letters are "EL" and I got her on the first of May, so it seemed an appropriate name.'

I found myself gazing at Harriet's pale skin and auburn hair and thought how very attractive she was but it wasn't just her appearance; she was bright, intelligent and fun to be with. I was aware that my feelings for her were very different from the way I had felt about Sarah. I very much hoped she might have some similar feelings for me but it seemed too much to hope for. My train of thought was suddenly interrupted by a return of the niggling doubt I had about whether or not I had told Harriet where Sarah lived. The more I thought about it the more certain I became that I hadn't. My first reaction was to forget about it but something inside me wouldn't let me and somewhat against my better judgement, I confronted her.

'Harriet, I'm sure I didn't tell you where Sarah lives. How do you know she lives near here?'

She paused as if trying to find the right words and for a few moments looked very uncomfortable which made me begin to feel guilty that I was pressing her on the subject.

'You're right, Justin, you didn't tell me. I know she lives near here because I followed you last night when you took her home. Please don't think I was spying on you but I wanted to know what was going on and I didn't entirely believe you when you said you'd finished with her. Please don't be annoyed with me. I know I shouldn't have followed you but I couldn't help it.'

'How did you know where to find me in order to be able to follow me?' I asked with a note of indignation.

'It was pure chance really. I was feeling a bit troubled and decided to go for a drive. I found myself heading towards your cottage and by pure chance I spotted you as you turned into Tunnel Road so I followed you. It was impulse – I didn't set out with the intention of following you and I very nearly ran into the back of you when you turned the corner and stopped outside Sarah's house. You wouldn't have been very happy with me if I had, would you? Anyway, at least I was left in no doubt that she wasn't very pleased with you from the way she slammed your car – she nearly turned it over.'

'So you now believe me when I say it's over between her and me?'

'Yes though the timing of the breakup wasn't exactly as you told me, was it?' she smiled as she said it and it didn't come over as an accusation.

'Not exactly but it is definitely over.' I was a little bit put out that she had followed me but, in the circumstances it was understandable particularly if it was true she hadn't planned it. I suppose I also wanted to consider it a good sign that she was sufficiently interested in me to want to follow me.

Before I had time to think any more about it my attention was taken by the sight of a yellow van in the distance. 'I think the AA might be here now,' I exclaimed. I was right and soon the cheery driver was towing my poor little car on to the back of his truck. It looked a sorry sight indeed.

'You made a bit of a mess of it,' he commented chirpily as he picked up some pieces of scrap metal that had become detached from the rest of the wreck and threw them nonchalantly onto the truck.

'You can say that again,' I groaned. 'Do you think it can be repaired or will it be written off?'

'It's not for me to say,' replied the AA driver 'but looking at it, I think it's doubtful if it would be economic to repair it. My instructions are to take it to Regal Motors at Sonnington and the insurance company's engineer will probably want to look at it in the next day or two, then someone will contact you to let you know what's been decided .'

Harriet sensed my dismay and took hold of my hand which I found very comforting. I felt that she was sharing my sadness as we stood and watched the AA truck disappear from view.

'Come on then,' she announced, 'let's get you home.'

I was a bit apprehensive about Harriet's driving in view of what I had heard and my nerves were somewhat frayed after the accident but I had to admit that her driving was flawless and very soon we were safely back at my cottage.

'Your driving's very good,' I declared with complete sincerity as she switched off the engine.

'You don't have to say that,' she replied though I sensed she was pleased to receive the compliment. I was, however, more than a bit disconcerted at her next statement.

'I ought to be wearing glasses really – I'm terribly short sighted; in fact I can't see much at all unless it's right under my nose. I hate wearing them though.'

'You really ought to if your eyesight's that bad.'

'I know; my mother's always on to me about it. I do wear them when I'm driving at night.'

'Oh, good!' I said teasingly. 'Perhaps in future when you intend going out in your car you would phone and let me know so that I can keep off the road.'

'You just said my driving was good,' she replied with a smile, clearly unoffended by my jibe.

'It was good but I'd still feel happier if you wore your glasses.'

She decided not to continue this line of conversation. 'Shall I make some coffee?' she enquired, changing the subject.

'That's a good idea; I'll come and help you.'

We went into the kitchen together though I'm sure she didn't need my help to make coffee, but I just wanted to be with her. There appeared to be something on her mind as she filled the kettle. 'It could be some time before you get your car sorted out,' she announced thoughtfully. 'You can borrow Ellie May in the meantime, if you'd like to.'

I was completely overwhelmed by the kindness of her offer.

'Harriet, that is very sweet of you but I couldn't possibly do that. You've only just got her and what are you going to do for transport?'

'I managed without one before; I don't really need a car. If I need to go somewhere I can always borrow my mother's.'

'I just don't know what to say. You hardly know me and you are offering to lend me your new car. It's just so incredibly generous; I'm completely blown away.'

'I know enough about you to know I can trust you to look after her and I would like to help.'

'I don't want to take her from you, Harriet. It's a wonderful gesture and I'm very flattered and honoured to think that you would trust me with her but I honestly couldn't. Tonight proved to me that any of us can be involved in an accident at any time, however careful we are; I couldn't live with myself if I damaged your car.'

'It's not likely to happen to you again so soon, I wouldn't think,' she responded, then a mischievous smile lit up her face. 'I know why you don't want to borrow her – it's because you don't want to be seen driving a little Morris 1000. Not the sort of image you want to project. You think you won't look so dashing and won't be so attractive to women.' As she spoke she gently prodded me in the ribs to emphasise the point.

'That's not it at all. In fact, right now there is only one woman I want to be attractive to and she's standing right in front of me.'

I felt myself being drawn towards her as I looked deep into her gorgeous blue eyes. My heart missed a beat when I realized she was looking at me with equal intensity and I was aware of a strange force making us interact with each other. I placed my hand gently on her shoulder and I felt a slight but unmistakeable response to my touch which encouraged me to go on. I stroked her hair and her perfume drifted over me. Her pale skin glowed and her eyes shone even brighter and clearer. I hesitated for a moment then I kissed her first on the cheek and then on her lips which were warm, inviting and very receptive.

As we moved apart after some seconds my first thought was whether I had gone too far too soon. My feelings for Harriet were developing strongly and rapidly and the last thing I wanted was to spoil things between us. When I looked back into her eyes, however, I felt there was a strangely enigmatic union between us and I realized that it had probably been present from the first moment we met.

'Can I see you again soon?' I asked earnestly.

'There's nothing I'd like more,' she whispered, 'but I have to go back to Southampton tomorrow and I shall be away for a week.'

CHAPTER THIRTY TWO

I had to walk to the surgery next morning. The weather was fine and I thought that the exercise would be good for me. In fact, I began to wonder why I didn't walk there more often instead of always taking my car. After all, it wasn't very far and I found that walking gave me an opportunity to think, without being distracted by the demands of driving. My mind was in a whirl anyway following the events that had taken place yesterday evening. I was naturally upset about smashing my car but this was completely overridden by the feeling of elation at the way my relationship with Harriet was progressing.

I had declined her offer to lend me her car because I felt it wouldn't be fair to deprive her of it so soon after she had obtained it. She was obviously thrilled about owning it and I was completely stunned when she offered so readily to let me borrow it. It was a completely and utterly selfless gesture and made me think that she must think a lot of me to make such an offer. I very much wanted to think that her response when I kissed her confirmed this perception.

When I arrived at the practice, Spencer was outside with a screwdriver in his hand attending to the doorknob, which a patient had reported as being loose. Dotty was running around looking most put out because the maintenance activities were preventing her from getting her usual morning walk. As soon as she saw me she appeared to brighten up and came over to let me stroke her. Spencer was surprised to see that I was on foot.

'Is this your idea of keeping fit, Justin?'

'Not exactly, Spencer; I crashed my car last night – I think it might be a write-off.'

'Oh bad luck,' he replied in a matter of fact tone of voice. 'It's a real nuisance when that happens; I've written off three or four in my time but it'll all get sorted eventually. I'm afraid I've got some rather sad news this morning; Balfour Mackean was found dead at the wheel of his car yesterday. He was out doing his house calls and suffered a heart attack. Fortunately he wasn't actually driving at the time; he must have felt ill and pulled off the road. He was found half way between here and Westport.'

'I'm really sorry to hear that; it's awful. I liked Balfour, he was a great character and his patients are certainly going to miss him. They all thought the world of him.'

'Yes they did. I shall miss him too; he and I used to go out for a pint together from time to time. I loved listening to the tales he used to tell me about his patients though I'm not convinced they were all true but he could spin a good yarn.'

'What's going to happen to his practice? He worked single-handed didn't he so his patients will be without a doctor at the moment?'

'I've no idea. I expect someone will come and take over. Are you registered with him?'

'Yes I am, though I've only seen him once professionally and that was when I went for an insurance medical.'

'I remember that. He rather put you through the mill, didn't he?'

'He did and I wasn't expecting it because you'd told me you didn't think the examination would be too searching; in fact it turned out to be quite the opposite.'

Spencer smiled at the memory. 'Good old Balfour. Luccombury won't be quite the same without him as the local doctor. I was also hoping we could resume our general anaesthetic sessions – I'd been meaning to contact him about it. Perhaps the new doctor will be willing to offer the same service.'

'I sincerely hope not, Spencer, but whether he does or not, you can count me out – I finished up in hospital thanks to that confounded gas machine.'

'Yes I know you did but that was your fault for not being more careful. You can't blame the machine.'

'Of course I blame the machine – it was faulty and leaking gas. Have you had it fixed yet?'

'No I haven't got around to it but I will. I'm still convinced that offering treatment under general anaesthetic could be a good money spinner for the practice.'

'Well don't expect me to get involved and don't ask me to help you repair the machine. I want nothing to do with it.'

'All right, all right, I get the message. Oh by the way, you'll be pleased to know that the dental company will be installing your new equipment later this week. They phoned up a few minutes ago.'

'That's great. I can't wait to start using it. Did they say what day they'd be coming?'

'No. They just didn't want to turn up and find it wasn't convenient for them to work. I said that the room is ready so they could come when they like. It will probably be Thursday or Friday, I suspect.'

'Thanks, Spencer, that's good news though I'm really sorry to hear about poor old Balfour.'

I left Spencer trying to sort out the problem with the doorknob though I gathered from his sudden expletive that things weren't exactly going to plan. Mrs Crossley was cleaning the stairs with the vacuum cleaner and I immediately wondered if she had yet seen her doctor and if so, how she'd got on. She appeared much less anxious than when she'd been searching for a diagnosis to her problem in Spencer's medical book though she looked slightly awkward when she saw me.

'I'm glad I've seen you, Mrs Crossley. How did you get on at the doctor's?'

'All right thank you, Justin.'

'So you haven't got cancer?'

'No.'

'That is good news; I told you it probably wouldn't be. I'm so pleased.'

'Yes. It was a great relief.'

'So you didn't have to go to the hospital for tests or anything?'

'No, it wasn't necessary.'

I didn't like to probe too much but it seemed a bit strange that the doctor could make such a quick and definite diagnosis on something which could have been potentially very serious. I was intrigued to know but wasn't quite sure what to say next. My hesitation prompted her to elaborate.

'I felt a bit stupid really, Justin.'

'Really, Mrs Crossley, I'm sure you had no reason at all to feel stupid. Passing blood can be very serious and needs to be investigated.'

'Ah well, it wasn't actually blood.'

'Wasn't it?'

'No. I told you I was going on to broccoli and beetroot?'

'I get it now – it was the beetroot?'

'That's right and the broccoli was adding to the symptoms. I think I probably overdid both of them. The doctor was very understanding but I felt such a fool.'

'It was an easy mistake to make but all's well that ends well; you'll know next time.'

'There won't be next time, I've given up the beetroot and the broccoli; I don't like the stuff anyway.'

I smiled and squeezed past her and the vacuum cleaner to get to my surgery. She didn't like people doing that as she was convinced it was unlucky to pass someone on the stairs but she didn't make a fuss about it on that occasion. Wendy was already in my surgery getting it ready for my first patient and she looked pensive and slightly melancholy. I assumed that Spencer had told her about Balfour MacKean.

'Yes, Spencer did tell me,' she exclaimed, 'how awful. I'm really sorry. I didn't actually know him but I think it's always sad when someone dies alone like that and it's a great shame that he didn't live to enjoy retirement.'

'I know what you mean but I think he loved his work and at least he didn't suffer or die a long and lingering death. Many people would say that it's a good way to go – but I agree; it's still very sad.

'Spencer's just told me that my new equipment is due to be installed this week and I'm really excited about that. We've still got a few minutes before my first patient is due, I'm just going downstairs to check something in the new surgery; I'll be back in a minute.'

Mrs Crossley had finished her cleaning and had packed away the vacuum cleaner so I didn't have to risk violating her superstition a second time. I was about to go downstairs when the front door opened and Spencer entered accompanied by a tall, slim, well-dressed gentleman whose sallow face and copious grey hair were familiar to me. I heard the man say 'the name's Hilary Husslebry – my close friends call me HH. I'm really a patient of Mr Derwent's.'

'Oh that doesn't matter,' I heard Spencer reply. 'You're a patient of the practice and I'm sure Mr Derwent won't mind if I take over your care from now on. I don't know how much he quoted you for the treatment but I think I ought to reassess the whole thing and we can discuss the cost when I've had time to formulate a proper treatment plan.'

'Well if you're sure, Padginton.'

'Quite sure. This type of work requires considerable experience, which of course I have. You'll be in safe hands with me.'

'I did think that Derwent was a bit of a whippersnapper so I'm somewhat relieved that I shall be getting the boss and not the apprentice.'

'Don't get me wrong; Mr Derwent is an excellent dentist but he's young and there's no substitute for experience. What time was your appointment with him?'

'Nine fifteen.'

'I already have a nine fifteen patient but I shouldn't be long with her– I'll fit you in immediately after.'

'You won't keep me waiting long will you, Padginton? I hate having my time wasted – I'm an extremely busy man, you know.'

'I fully understand, Mr Husslebry. I hate to keep patients waiting and I always avoid it whenever possible but I if you could bear with me this morning, I'll make sure that in future you are seen on time.'

'Very well, Padginton, but be as quick as you can.'

Spencer saw me on the stairs and looked embarrassed because he realized that I had caught him in the act of poaching one of my patients. What he didn't know was that I was delighted to be getting rid of Mr Husslebry who was always extremely difficult and unpleasant. Nothing was ever right for him; he questioned everything I did and demanded an explanation for every decision I made. He also expected to be seen exactly on time and would not tolerate being kept waiting, which was sometimes unavoidable. Spencer was most welcome to him and would, I felt sure, live to rue the day that he invited him to transfer from me to him.

Spencer obviously felt awkward about it and came to speak to me. 'I hope you don't mind my taking over Mr Husslebry's treatment, Justin. It's just that these elderly, upper middle class patients tend to be very wary of young and relatively inexperienced practitioners. I know that, in your case, there's no justification but that's the way they see things I'm afraid. All young dentists have to endure this; I did myself when I first started in general practice.'

'So it wasn't your idea to get him to transfer to you because you knew that he was a private patient who needed quite a lot of work done and you thought it might be quite lucrative to have him on your books?' I smiled as I said it to let Spencer know that I bore no malice over the transfer.

'Of course not, Justin; you know I'd never do that,' Spencer replied unconvincingly.

'Well I wish you luck with him. Frankly, I found him a pain in the backside.'

'That's because he didn't fully trust you for the reasons I've just mentioned so it's better for everyone if I treat him from now on. I'm so pleased we've sorted this amicably. I would hate you to think I'd steal one of your patients.'

Because Mr Husslebry's appointment with me had been at nine fifteen, when the time arrived I was free to make myself a cup of coffee and sit down with the newspaper. I sat down in the office enjoying my few minutes of relaxation when I heard something of a commotion downstairs.

'Are you going to be much longer, Padginton?' demanded Mr Husslebry who was banging furiously on Spencer's surgery door with his head up against the glass panel, peering in to see what Spencer was doing. 'I told you I'm a very busy man and I can't afford to be kept waiting.'

Spencer stopped what he was doing and emerged from his surgery with a bright red face. He was clearly very irate but struggled to maintain his decorum. 'I told you I would be a bit late, Mr Husslebry. You knew I already had a lady booked in for treatment at nine fifteen and you agreed to wait, now please take a seat in the waiting room and I'll be with you just as soon as I can.'

'I didn't know you'd keep me waiting as long as this,' Mr Husslebry protested.

'I'm going as fast as I can and it is only nine twenty,' Spencer insisted.

'Not by my watch it isn't: I make it after twenty-five past.'

'Then your watch is wrong!' Spencer barked and disappeared back into his surgery leaving Mr Husslebry standing in the hall looking extremely indignant. He didn't return to the waiting room but stood with his face glued to the glass panel watching and assessing Spencer's rate of progress with his female patient. Every few seconds he would look again at his watch and mutter to himself. I chuckled and returned to my coffee and newspaper thinking that Spencer might one day think that it might have been better if there hadn't been a glass panel in his new surgery door.

CHAPTER THIRTY THREE

I rather gathered that Spencer had quite a tough time with Mr Husselbry who was very annoyed about being kept waiting in spite of the fact he had been warned that he couldn't be seen on time on this occasion. He was totally unreasonable about it, as I knew he would be, and I got the feeling that Spencer was beginning to wonder exactly what he had let himself in for by taking over his treatment. I had very little sympathy because Spencer had been very eager to poach him from me when he thought he could make some money out of him and my feelings were that if the whole thing turned sour, he only had himself to blame. Although my morning had not been entirely trouble-free, I couldn't help thinking it would have been a lot worse if I had been forced to endure Mr Husselbry's bad temper and his incessant moaning about the treatment I was providing for him.

I was sitting at my desk writing up record cards when Spencer came into my surgery looking very solemn. 'Have you a moment please, Justin? I'd like you to take a look at one of my patients and give me your opinion. It's Mr Jolly who's been a patient of mine for many years. He's never had much trouble in the past but recently I've noticed a very dramatic deterioration in his gum condition and I feel fairly sure there must be an underlying medical condition. Will you have a look and tell me what you think?'

I followed Spencer downstairs to his surgery and he introduced me to his patient.

I shook hands with him. 'Hello, Mr Jolly,'

'That's me. Jolly by name and jolly by nature,' he replied with a grin.

'Do you mind if my colleague, Mr Derwent, has a look at your gums,' Spencer requested.

'My goodness,' Mr Jolly chortled. 'What have I done to deserve all this attention?'

Spencer provided the answer. 'I'm a bit concerned about the state of your gums and the fact that they seem to have suddenly become very inflamed and I want Mr Derwent to see what he thinks about them, if that's all right with you.'

'That's all right with me. Be my guest, Mr Derwent.'

It was immediately apparent that his gums were red and inflamed. They looked sore and bled very easily. 'There isn't any calculus or plaque on the teeth to cause irritation,' I observed, 'and you say the condition developed quickly and recently, Spencer, so there must be an underlying cause.'

'That's what I thought, Justin, but I thought I'd let you have a look. Mr Jolly, we don't know why your gums have suddenly become sore like this but there's obviously a reason for it. Have you noticed any other changes? Do you feel unwell?'

'No not really. I've felt a bit tired recently but I put it down to the fact I'm not getting any younger. Apart from that, nothing, though it's true that my gums have suddenly started bleeding when I brush my teeth and they never used to.'

'Well,' Spencer continued, 'if you don't mind, I'd like to refer you to the hospital so that they can find out what's causing the problem.'

'Hospital, Mr Padginton? I don't want to go to the hospital,' he protested in his broad Dorset accent. 'Surely that's not necessary; can't you give me some tablets or mouthwash or something to clear it up?'

'I'll give you some mouthwash which might help but that's not the complete answer, I'm afraid. There could be an underlying medical problem – it might be nothing – but I think we ought to find out.'

'Medical problem? I've never had a day's illness in my life; I can't believe there's anything wrong with me.'

'Perhaps there isn't, Mr Jolly and I hope you're right but I really think we need to find out why your gums have suddenly started bleeding.'

217

'Well what could it be, Mr Padginton?'

'As I said, it might be nothing at all,' Spencer replied soothingly, 'but you could be suffering from a medical condition that is causing your gums to become sore and if you are, then the sooner it's diagnosed and treated the better.'

'What sort of condition?'

'I can't say, Mr Jolly because I don't know. All I'm saying is that it would be advisable to get it checked out in case it's something that requires treatment.'

'You've got me worried now, Mr Padginton.'

'I'll write to the hospital today and get them to give you an appointment as soon as possible so they can sort this out for you. In the meantime, try not to worry.'

'I don't like the look of it,' Spencer sighed as soon as Mr Jolly had left. 'I hope it turns out to be something simple.'

'You were right to refer him though, Spencer. It's lucky that he comes for regular check-ups and that you spotted the change in his gum condition. If it is something serious there's a good chance it can be diagnosed and treated early, thanks to you. He obviously hasn't felt ill enough to see a doctor about it yet and it could be some time before he does, by which time the condition, if it is a serious one, would be much more advanced.'

'I'll write to the hospital right away,' said Spencer with urgency in his voice.

I returned to my surgery hoping that Mr Jolly was not suffering from a serious medical condition but at least, thanks to Spencer's perceptiveness he would receive the necessary treatment quickly. It made me think that being a dentist was not just about fixing people's teeth; there were times when the role acquired an additional purpose which was in many ways more important.

I was feeling slightly apprehensive because my next patient was Mrs Newman who was coming to have her permanent crowns fitted. The technician had done a wonderful job in making the crowns look natural with lots of character. They were very white which was what Mrs Newman wanted; they were also very large.

Although it was obviously a big day for Mrs Newman and one she had been looking forward to for some time, she certainly hadn't dressed for the occasion. She was wearing a faded old tartan dress which looked old enough to have belonged to her mother. Her hair hadn't seen a comb or a brush since she got out of bed and her face didn't have a trace of make-up.

'They look even better than the temporary crowns, Mr Derwent.'

'Yes, the technician has done a good job but are you absolutely certain they're what you want? Once they're fitted it won't be easy to alter them. Look at the length, I personally still think they're too big but you seem to be sure you want them like that.'

'Yes I do, I'm certain of it.'

I was very tempted to stick them on with temporary cement in case she changed her mind later on but as she seemed so convinced they were right I went ahead and fixed them permanently. As she left, I couldn't help thinking it was all a big mistake. She looked all teeth and I was convinced that when her friends and family gave their opinion she would be forced to admit she'd got it wrong. My greatest fear was that she would ask for the crowns to be removed. I suggested making a follow up appointment which I would face with a certain amount of trepidation.

CHAPTER THIRTY FOUR

I hadn't seen Ephraim for over a week. Ordinarily, I saw him most days attending to his pigeons, either when I left for work in the morning or when I got home in the evening but lately there had been no sign of him. Then it occurred to me that he must be deliberately avoiding me because of his tooth problem. I decided to seek him out.

I knocked on his door and Nellie's bark let me know he was at home. She went everywhere with him so if she was at home – so was he, but it was some time before the door opened and he appeared. He looked absolutely awful. His eyes were red and puffy and suggested he hadn't been sleeping properly and his face was still visibly swollen.

'Thought 'ee'd come and find I sooner or later,' was his opening remark. I'm not sure if he had been dreading seeing me or hoping I would track him down; possibly a mixture of both. 'Better come in,' he grunted.

Ephraim's housekeeping left a lot to be desired at the best of times but this time his kitchen was an absolute shambles with every square inch of horizontal surface piled high with cups, plates, saucepans, empty tins of beans and dog food, and beer bottles.

'How's the tooth?' I enquired. I had a good idea that it was still giving him a lot of trouble though I doubted if he would give me an honest answer. Surprisingly, he opened up and confirmed that he'd had a rough time over the past few days.

'Don't mention it; I've just about 'ad as much as I can take from it. Tried to pull bugger out wi' a pair o' pliers last night.'

'And did you manage it?'

'No, couldn't get hold on it; it's so broken down. I don't see 'ow you'd be able to get 'old neither so I didn't reckon there was any point in coming to see about it.'

'Didn't the antibiotics help?'

'Fer a time but they soon wore off, then 'twere just as bad. Can't 'ee give I some stronger pills?'

'It really needs to come out.'

The expression on his face was enough to tell me that the idea of having it extracted terrified him. 'But if there's nothin' to get 'old on, 'ee won't be able to, will 'ee?'

'I'll be able to remove it for you, Ephraim. I'm sure it won't be that difficult.'

'But 'ow? I don't think 'tis possible.'

'Let me worry about that. You just come to the surgery at five o'clock tomorrow and I'll deal with it for you.'

The look of fear in his eyes was beginning to turn to panic. 'I couldn't, Justin, I der hate anythin' like that. Just give me more pills, I'm sure it'll get better given time; most things do if yer wait long enough.'

'Not necessarily and it's not doing your general health any good either. Why suffer like this, Ephraim, when the whole thing can be put right for good in a matter of minutes?'

'It's easy for you to say.'

'There's really nothing to worry about; you'll be amazed how easy it will be.'

He wasn't at all convinced. 'Can't you give me gas – put I to sleep?'

'I can't do that, I'm afraid. We don't do it anymore.' I hoped that word had not reached him about Spencer's excursion into the world of general anaesthesia but I overlooked the fact that he had a good memory.

'You der do it. I know that because you finished up in hospital after gassing yourself.'

'You're right, I did, but that was the first and last time we used the machine – it's not safe so we stopped using it. You'll have to go to hospital if you want to be put to sleep.'

'No fear,' he snapped, 'yer won't get I in there. Once they get their 'ands on you, you be lucky to get out.'

'Well then, Ephraim, it will have to be an injection in your gum. It'll be fine – you won't feel a thing and the tooth will be out in a flash.'

'I can't do it, Justin. I hate to admit it but I'm just too scared – there, I've said it now. I tried to hide it from you but the idea of going and having it yanked out terrifies me.'

'I've known all along that you're scared – you didn't do a very good job of hiding it from me. I also know that you've been avoiding me for the past week but you must be desperate to try to extract it yourself with a pair of pliers. You're going to have to face it but it won't be half as bad as you think.'

'Can't you give I something to calm I down before I der come? I'd need something pretty strong 'cos even whisky won't work.'

'I can give you some tranquillizers. If you come to the surgery first thing tomorrow morning I'll write a prescription for you, then you can get them from the chemist and take some before you come to see me at five o'clock.'

'Are you sure they'll work? I've never taken tranquillizers afore.'

'They'll work all right. You won't have a care in the world after taking two of those tablets; you'll be absolutely amazed. Now try to get some sleep tonight and don't worry about a thing. If you meet me at half past eight tomorrow morning we can walk to the surgery together.'

Much to my surprise, Ephraim was waiting for me outside his cottage when I left for work next morning. He didn't say a lot and I noticed that he was walking a bit unsteadily. When I got nearer to him and smelled the alcohol on his breath I realized he had already been on the whisky. 'I wouldn't drink any more alcohol today if I were you, Ephraim, it doesn't mix very well with the tablets I'm going to give you.'

'I need something to help sooth my nerves, Justin.'

'What I suggest is that you stay off the drink for the rest of the day but you can take one of the tablets after lunch to help steady you and then you can take two more about four o'clock before coming to see me at five. Have you got that?'

'I think so. I sure hope they der work 'cos right now I feel as bad as if I were goin' to meet my executioner.'

There were already two other patients in the waiting room when we arrived at the practice and Ephraim did a marvellous job of unsettling them. First he sat down for about half a minute then he

222

started pacing backwards and forwards, puffing, blowing and grunting before declaring his terror to them.

'There's really nothing to fear, old chap,' I heard one of the patients say in a vain attempt to offer reassurance. 'Dentistry is virtually painless these days; you hardly feel anything.'

Unfortunately, his words were lost on Ephraim who suddenly slumped to the floor, clutching his chest, wheezing and gasping, 'I'm having a heart attack,' he screamed, 'get help.'

I was on the point of delivering his prescription when I heard his cries and as soon as I saw that his breathing was rapid and shallow I immediately suspected he was suffering a panic attack so I grabbed a paper bag from the kitchen and got him to breathe into it. Fortunately, my spot diagnosis was correct and soon his breathing slowed and he became calmer.

'Ooh,' he groaned, 'I reckoned I was a gonner just then.'

'You've just got yourself worked up, Ephraim. You need to slow down your breathing.'

'So I'm not having a heart attack? I was sure I was. I said to myself "Ephraim, old son, this is it, yer number's up".'

'No you're all right but you must try to calm down. Sit here for a while and take some deep breaths and when you feel well enough, I suggest you walk slowly to the chemist's and get these tablets. Perhaps it would be a good idea to take one straightaway.' I handed him the prescription.

'Shall I still take one after lunch and two at four o'clock?' he asked.

I pondered for a moment. It was always difficult to predict exactly how people would react to medication because some needed a higher dosage than others in order to achieve the desired effect and Ephraim was an unknown quantity. I thought he would probably need a strong dose to overcome his nerves but I didn't want to overdo the tranquillization.

'I suggest you take one as soon as you get them and one after lunch and see how you get on. If you feel less anxious then perhaps you only need to take one tablet at four o'clock, though you can take two if you need to but don't take any more than that and don't drink any whisky with them.'

He was a pathetic sight sitting on the edge of a chair in the waiting room with a look of impending doom etched upon his unshaven face. I felt sorry for him because he couldn't help being

223

scared and I was well aware that nothing I could say to him would ease his feelings. I thought perhaps the fear of dying might have outweighed his dread of having his tooth extracted and for a very short time I think it did but now that he knew he wasn't dying, his thoughts returned to his tooth.

I didn't see him leave so I have no idea how long he stayed in the waiting room and I wondered if he would turn up at five o'clock. The hour arrived and greatly to my amazement so did he and made quite a dramatic entrance. Wendy happened to be in the hall at the time and heard a dull thud against the door. When she opened it, Ephraim stumbled forwards groping at the door frame for support and with Wendy's assistance, just managed to avoid falling headlong on to the rug at the bottom of the stairs. His eyes were glazed and staring and he was mumbling incoherently. I shall never know how he had managed to walk from his cottage to the surgery because, at the moment, he was having great difficulty just standing without being propped up and he was exuding whisky fumes, powerful enough to make your eyes water, with every exhalation.

'Justin, can you come and help?' Wendy called out whilst she hung on to his arm trying to steady him as he swayed from side to side, almost pulling her down with him. I ran down the stairs and grabbed his other arm. Together we managed to steer him towards a chair in the entrance hall.

'I can't face it, Justin,' he muttered in slurred tones. 'I can't face it.' He looked towards me but his eyes didn't focus.

'We'll never get him upstairs, Wendy. Is Spencer still in his surgery?'

'No, he finished with his last patient half an hour ago. He's in his workshop,' Wendy replied.

'Then let's put him in Spencer's surgery. Next week at this time mine should be downstairs too but as it isn't at the moment, I'll have to use Spencer's. I'm sure he won't mind in the circumstances.'

'I shouldn't think he will,' Wendy agreed. We hoisted Ephraim out of the chair and shuffled him into Spencer's dental chair. His legs were crumpling beneath him and we had to support his entire weight which was considerably greater than I would have expected. Wendy and I were both exhausted by the time we had him safely seated.

'I can't face it, Justin, jus' leave me alone. I don' want 'ee to take out my tooth — 'tas stopped hurting now. I'm sure 'twill be all right if 'ee were to leave it be now.'

224

'We can't leave it, Ephraim. It has to come out.'

Ephraim continued to ramble. 'Don' hurt no more. I can't see no good reason fer takin' it out now; 'tis fine now – good as new. I don't think I need trouble 'ee no more. I'm real grateful for all 'ee's done but I'll be on my way now an' not take up any more o' yer time.' He tried to get out of the chair but his coordination failed him completely and with Wendy's help he slipped back down on to the seat.

'He obviously been drinking,' said Wendy, 'presumably he's taken some tranquillizers as well.'

'Quite a few by the look of him,' I replied. 'How many tablets have you taken, Ephraim?'

His brow furrowed as he tried desperately to be coherent. 'Just a few. Not too sure really; can't remember now.'

'Have you got them with you?'

He fumbled in each pocket in turn and finally produced the bottle which he handed to me with a trembling hand. I counted the tablets and on the assumption he had swallowed the ones that were missing from the full prescription, I established he had taken six which together with whisky amounted to fairly hefty knock-out combination, though not enough to cause major concern.

Wendy was striving to prevent him from slumping down in the chair and became alarmed when he suddenly threw back his head, rolled his eyes and then let out a groan and appeared to lose consciousness. 'Oh my God, he's dead,' she screamed.

A quick check of his carotid pulse confirmed he was in fact still with us, though his heart rate was somewhat slow. I could also see that he was still breathing. 'He's not dead; he's just passed out, which is hardly surprising in view of the cocktail of drugs and whisky he's taken today. He'll be all right.'

'What are you going to do with him now?' asked Wendy still looking very concerned.

'I'm going to take out his tooth. That's what he's here for and that's what I'm going to do. Whilst he's in this state, he's not likely to put up any opposition.'

Wendy said nothing but I don't think she was convinced it was a good idea. However, she handed me a syringe and I injected some lignocaine to anaesthetise his tooth though I doubt if it was really necessary. The persistent infection around the tooth had loosened it over a period of time and it was actually quite easy to extract it. Ephraim's fear that I wouldn't be able to get hold of it turned out to be groundless, as I had predicted, and I was able to slide the beaks of a pair of narrow forceps between the tooth and the gum and gain a firm hold on the root which, fortunately, was not too broken down. The whole procedure took just a few minutes. Now I had to decide what to do with Ephraim. He was clearly in no state to take himself home.

'Ephraim, can you hear me?' I shouted to him.

'Uh? What? Where am I? I can't face it, Justin, just leave me be,' came the garbled reply.

'It's out, Ephraim. Your tooth's out.'

'I can't face it, please don't take it out. I jus' want to go 'ome. It'll get better in time if you leave it alone. I don't think it needs to come out.'

'Ephraim, listen to me. Your tooth's out, look it's here.' I held it up for him to see and for a moment his face lit up but I don't think my words really sank in and he couldn't believe what he was seeing. He probably thought he was dreaming or hallucinating. His eyes appeared to be trying to focus for a few moments then they closed again and he drifted back into unconsciousness.

'What are you going to do with him?' queried Wendy. 'You haven't got a car at the moment, have you? Shall I ask Spencer to take him home?'

'No, don't trouble Spencer; I'll phone for a taxi.'

By the time the taxi arrived, Ephraim had rallied round to some extent and was beginning to accept that his tooth had been removed.

'I can't believe it, Justin, brilliant, fantastic. There was absolutely nothing to it. I can honestly say I never felt a thing.' His speech was still very slurred and he continued swaying from side to side but the sheer elation of having come through the procedure seemed to be helping him fight off the effects of the tranquillizers and alcohol – for the moment. I felt sure that very soon the stress and lack of sleep would catch up with him and he would sink into a semi-comatose state. I hoped I could get him home before that happened and I decided to go with him in the taxi.

The taxi driver helped me get him onto his sofa after clearing it of old newspapers and beer cans. There was no way we could get him upstairs to bed but he looked comfortable enough and I covered him with a blanket. Nellie jumped up beside him and took over the job of looking after him. Throughout the evening I checked on him every hour to see that he was all right. I was prepared to make him some tea or coffee or get him something to eat but he didn't wake up at all so at ten o'clock I turned out the lights, locked his door and left him to sleep.

I was amazed next morning to find him up and about when I left for work. What was even more remarkable was that he looked perfectly fresh and completely unaffected by his ordeal. Nellie, on the other hand was lying with her head on her paws looking as if she'd had a rough night. 'Mornin', Justin,' he called out to me with a smug grin. 'Nothin' to it. Don't know why folk der get themselves all worked up 'bout comin' to see you fellas. Mind 'ee, I have to admit you were brilliant. Credit where credit's due is what I always say.'

'Thank you, Ephraim; I told you it would be easy but you didn't believe me.'

'Arr, 'tweren't that, Justin, but 'tis a long while since I set foot inside a dentist's like and yer sort o' gets out o' practice.'

'So now we've broken the ice, you'll come and let me sort out the rest of your teeth, will you? There are quite a few others that could play up in the same way.'

Ephraim suddenly looked less confident. 'Well, let's not be too hasty, we der need to let this settle first. Could take a while but per'aps I'll think about it later on.'

'I think you should. Anyway, I suggest you take things easy for a day or two – you're on the crest of a wave now but you've been though a lot in the past couple of weeks and your body needs to recover.'

'I'll bear that in mind. Now I'll go and feed my pigeons.'

CHAPTER THIRTY FIVE

I wasn't feeling particularly happy when I arrived home from work that evening because the insurance company had telephoned me during the afternoon to tell me that the damage to my car was beyond economic repair. In other words, it was a write-off. I was naturally upset because I liked the car but on the other hand, as the damage was so extensive I feared it would never be quite the same again even if they did manage to repair it. So now I had to go out and find another one which I intended to do as soon as I had an opportunity.

It started raining whilst I was walking home so I was now wet as well as depressed about my car. Ephraim greeted me before I had time to disappear through my front door; I gathered he had been waiting for me. 'Awri then, Justin? 'ad a good day?' he called out.

'Not too bad thanks, Ephraim. How about you?'

'Yer, t'were a good day. Went to the Barrel today. 'ee know it?'

'The Barrel? No I don't know it.'

' 'tis an old pub out in Marshwood Vale. "Cider Barrel" really, but we know it as "The Barrel". Used to go there a lot but I bain't bin fer nye on a month 'cos o' my tooth. I met up wi' me ol' mates, Giles, Saul, Jarvey an'Jake. 'ee'll be pleased to know I've bin drummin' up some business fer 'ee. Told en 'bout my tooth. They wouldn't believe I'd 'ad it out to begin wi'. "Never", they said. I 'ad to show en the 'ole wi' the blood in it before they'd accept 'twere true. They were staggered. "That's real brave" they said 'cos theyse like I used to be, scared stiff.'

'So you aren't scared any more then, Ephraim?'

'Told en; bain't nothin' to it an' I didn't even feel it cum out . When 'ee told me 'twere out I couldn't believe it – marvellous. Can 'onestly say I never felt a thing. Mind 'ee, credit where credit's due, I told en 'ee were fantastic. They were so impressed they said they thought they'd cum and give 'ee a try – get their teeth sorted out like 'cos I know Jarvey's 'ad toothache a time or two but were too afeared to do anythin' 'bout it.'

'Yes, thank you for the recommendation, Ephraim. I'll look forward to seeing them.'

I tried to sound enthusiastic but I was thinking that I sincerely hoped I wouldn't have the pleasure of seeing them professionally. The last thing I needed was four new patients with the same aversion to dentistry as Ephraim but I also knew from experience that it was most unlikely they would actually seek treatment unless driven to do so by prolonged and unbearable pain. The local scrumpy undoubtedly had the potential to give them the courage to make all sorts of pledges but I was pretty sure they would feel very differently when stone-cold sober.

'They zed they'd come over and get themselves sorted in the next day or two. I reckon I should be on commission – drumming up business for 'ee like that.'

'Yes, thank you, Ephraim. You did tell them they'll need to make appointments? They can't just turn up and expect to be seen straightaway.'

'Well no, I never thought. Can't 'ee just fit 'em in t'ave a look, like? Won't take long to do that.'

'I won't have time to fit in four of them all at once. If you see them again you need to tell them to phone up and make appointments, not just turn up unannounced. In any case, I doubt if they'll come; they said they would when you were in the pub but I expect their courage will fail them when it comes to the crunch.'

'Oh, doan' reckon,' said Ephraim confidently. 'They were mighty impressed that I wer' able to go through it 'cos they knew 'ow afeared I was. They zed if I cud do it, they cud too.'

I left him muttering to himself that he thought it was wonderful how he had managed to overcome his fear and face having his tooth extracted. He was quite proud of himself and I could just imagine how he would have boasted to his friends about his achievement. I very much doubted if he had told them he was completely zonked out on tranquillisers and whisky to the point of being completely oblivious to the whole procedure. In fact I felt sure he would not have admitted to them that he had needed to take tranquillizers.

I just wanted to get myself something to eat and sit down and unwind. I had bought a newspaper on my way home with the intention of looking at advertisements for second hand cars. Now I knew that I wouldn't be getting my little sports car repaired, the search for a replacement must begin in earnest – I had been without a car for too long already.

My evening meal was nothing special as I had failed to stick to my resolution to plan ahead and shop regularly for food so it had to be baked beans, cheese and tomatoes on toast because that was all I had in the house. Fortunately, I was so hungry I could have eaten anything and if there had been a more appetizing choice available to me it would have had to be something that could be prepared very quickly. I piled the food on to a plate and drew up a chair with the intention of reading the paper whilst eating. I had barely eaten enough to take the edge off my appetite when there was a loud knock at the door. 'Damn,' I said to myself, 'I really don't want to see any visitors at this very moment. Who the devil can it be?' I put down my knife and fork and suddenly the thought occurred to me that it might be Harriet. She was the one person in the world I would be pleased to see though when I last saw her she told me she would be in Southampton all week so it seemed unlikely that it would be her. But she had Ellie May now so she was quite mobile and it was just possible she had taken it upon herself to come and surprise me. My spirits lifted at the thought and I moved towards the door more swiftly. Sadly, I was to be disappointed; it wasn't her and when I saw the four grubby, unshaven, gumbooted countrymen standing there in the rain, my heart sank. I knew immediately who they were and what they'd come for.

'Mr Derwent?' enquired the shortest and roundest of the four.

'That's right,' I replied.

'We be real pleased to meet 'ee. We be friends of ole Ephraim and 'e's bin tellin' us 'ow you took out 'is tooth wi' out 'im feelin' nothin'. Dead easy 'e said 'twere; nothin' to it at all so we thought we'd cum an' get sorted out ourselves, cos we've all 'ad a bit o' tooth

230

trouble at odd times like. None o' us 'ave a reg'lar dentist, an' till Ephraim told us about 'ee we all said we'd rather suffer than go to one but Ephraim said 'twere so easy we should come and see 'ee right away, so 'ere we be.'

The smell of cider was overpowering and I quickly reached the conclusion that they must have stayed in the pub until they had drunk themselves into a state of alcohol-induced bravado. 'I don't work here,' I began, 'this is where I live and I finished working at half past five. You'll need to come to the surgery if you want treatment but you'll need to make appointments first.'

'Ephraim said 'ee'd see us,' replied the eldest member of the group looking quite crestfallen.

'I'm not saying I won't see you but I can't see you now. I suggest you phone the practice tomorrow and arrange some appointments.'

'We've sort of wound ourselves up to face comin' like and we'd hoped 'ee could see us straightaway. Ephraim said 'e felt sure 'ee would.'

'I'm sorry but Ephraim has misled you. I haven't got the equipment or the facilities to see you here; telephone the surgery tomorrow and make some appointments.'

'Can't 'ee take us to the surgery now and sort us out like? Save us comin' back.'

'I'm afraid I can't. The surgery is closed until nine o'clock tomorrow. After six o'clock in the evening it stops being a dental surgery and becomes Mr Padginton's home. I'm not prepared to disturb him and in any case I haven't got a nurse to help me at this time in the evening.'

''ee won't need no nurse,' said the little fat one, 'Giles can do that for 'ee; 'e were real good when 'e 'elped vet deliver Jim Wangle's calf last yer.'

'That's not quite the same as dental nursing,' I pointed out, beginning to feel slightly edgy. I realised that Ephraim had led them to believe they could just drop in on me and I would attend to their teeth straightaway. I also realised that it wasn't going to be easy to get rid of them without acceding to their request.

'I'm very sorry to disappoint you, gentlemen but I really cannot take you to the surgery this evening and as I can't treat you here, please do as I say and phone up tomorrow to make some appointments.'

The four of them looked completely thwarted and it was hard to believe they could really be so upset about not being able to get their teeth seen to, particularly as they were all supposed to be terrified of dentists and hadn't seen one for many years. I was hoping they would accept my last statement as the final word but they weren't finished yet. The one who I had worked out to be Giles moved closer to me and after a furtive glance all round to see if anyone else was in earshot, whispered, 'We'll see thee awri.' He winked at me as he said it and the other three nodded in agreement.

'I'm afraid it's still no,' I replied stubbornly. Their body language suggested they were still not prepared to give up and none of them gave any indication that he was about to back away. I decided that I needed to apply a bit of psychology to the situation.

'Gentlemen, you must realise that I've had a hard day today and I'm tired which means I probably wouldn't have the strength to take out your teeth even if I wanted to. Ephraim's tooth came out without any trouble because it was loose; you could have taken it out with your fingers really, but it's a completely different matter when the tooth isn't loose and you all look to me as if your teeth will be set in concrete. Do you know, you might find it hard to believe but I can tell just by looking at someone, how difficult it would be to take out their teeth? It's a skill that dentists develop.'

'That be right?' gasped the tall one in amazement, 'that's fantastic. Ephraim said 'ee were right clever.'

'Sometimes,' I continued, 'I have to put my knee against the patient's chest to hold them down in the chair whilst I pull; otherwise I would lift them clean out of the chair.'

'No!' Giles gulped, looking slightly less enthusiastic about getting his dental treatment. 'I don't believe it, 'ee don't look strong enough to do that.'

'Don't be fooled by my slight appearance. Once I get going and I'm determined to get a tooth out my strength seems to intensify until I've managed it.'

'I've 'eard that sort o' thing can 'appen,' said the fourth member of the group who until now had remained quiet. 'Seems 'ee der get extra powers from somewhere just as 'ee can run twice as fast as normal when a bull's chasing 'ee like.'

'Yes, it's a bit like that,' I conceded. 'Anyway, I can tell just by looking at you four that I would have a terrible struggle trying to take out a tooth on any of you so there's no way I could treat all of you this evening, I'm just too tired. You'd need to come to see me first thing in the morning when I'm fresh.'

'But the pubs don' open till 'leven.'

'It would have to be nine o'clock – half past at the latest.'

'Don't know 'bout that,' said Giles. 'Don't think that'd fit in with our daily routine.'

'Well think about it and phone up tomorrow to make some appointments. I'll need to know when you're coming so that I can get an early night the night before. I shall need every ounce of strength I can muster to deal with you four as I can see that it's going to be real tussle to get your teeth out.'

'Ephraim said 'twere easy,' said the little one, looking distinctly alarmed.

'His was, but yours will be a different kettle of fish altogether.' I watched as the air of confidence they had when they arrived ebbed rapidly away from them. The fact that the effects of the local cider were beginning to wear off accelerated the rate at which this occurred. They turned and retreated from my door muttering to each other. I couldn't make out what they were saying and the Dorset dialect added to my lack of understanding.

CHAPTER THIRTY SIX

Ephraim was in his garden again next morning when I left for work. Now that his tooth had been dealt with, he no longer needed to avoid me and I had the feeling he had missed being able to talk to me and intended to make up for it now. 'Marnen, Justin,' he shouted.

'Good morning, Ephraim.'

'I understan' my mates came to visit 'ee last night; thought 'ee would see en t'ave their teeth done like if they came down 'ere.'

'I know, but I couldn't do anything for them at that time in the evening and they'll need to make appointments if they want treatment.'

'I think they might be changin' their minds 'bout that after 'ee told en their teeth'd be set in concrete an' 'ee'd 'ave to pull so 'ard 'ee'd lift en out o' the chair,' he chuckled.

'Yes they did seem a bit worried when I told them that,' I agreed.

'Did 'ee mean it?'

'Without looking in their mouths I couldn't really be sure but they're all tough looking characters and their teeth could be difficult to extract.'

'I'm glad 'ee never told me that afore I 'ad mine done.'

'You let me examine yours and I could see that it had been infected for a long time and the infection had helped to loosen it. It's possible the same thing has happened with your friends but I thought I'd paint the worst picture so they wouldn't be surprised if I gave them a bad time. Do you think they'll come back?'

'Very much doubt it,' he replied thoughtfully, 'scared off, I reckon. I thought I were doin' 'ee a favour – drummin' up business like.'

'I appreciate the thought, Ephraim, but people with a deep fear of dentistry are never easy and to have four of them descend upon me all at once is something I could probably live without.'

'Thought 'ee'd be pleased,' Ephraim retorted sulkily. 'Anyway, 'ows the car getting' on?'

'It's a write off, I'm afraid. I shall have to buy another one.'

'I der know just the man 'ee needs to see.'

'I think you've told me about him, Ephraim. He specializes in buying up old wrecks and putting them back on the road, very cheaply?'

'Noah, I don't mean 'e; this one's real respectable like, though more expensive – Vessey's 'is name.'

'Is that his Christian name?'

'I reckon so.'

'It's an unusual name.'

'Ay, 'tis. Any'ow 'e der run the garage out at Kittlewake, not far from 'ere. 'Tis on Lyme Regis road – 'ee can't miss it 'cos there be cars everywhere; the garage is overflowin' wi' en an' they stretch right down th'road. Everybody knows Vessey, 'e's mad on cars and took over some time back from 'is father who'd been there for years. Got a good reputation though; 'ee can trust Vessey not to swindle 'ee. Matter o' fact I bumped into 'e in Sonnington yesterday – we 'ad a good old natter 'cos I 'adn't seen 'im for some time. '

'I'll go and see if he's got anything I might be interested in as soon as I can but without a car it's difficult,' I said, hoping that Ephraim might offer to give me a lift out there but he didn't.

'Tell 'im ol' Ephraim sent 'ee an' 'e'll see thee awri.'

I asked Spencer if he knew Vessey and Kittlewake Garage.

'Everyone around here knows Vessey – he's a good chap with a first class reputation. He's got a lot of old bangers for sale but he does have some good stuff as well. He's completely reliable and will want you to be happy with whatever you buy. If I wanted a modern car, which I don't, but if I did, I'd have no hesitation in buying one from him.'

'That's a pretty good recommendation. I think I'll go and see if he's got anything that interests me but without a car it's difficult for me to get there.' I was hoping that maybe Spencer would be more obliging than Ephraim had been with regards to offering me a lift. Unfortunately, he had other plans.

'I'd take you there, Justin, but Daphne and I are going out for the evening straight after work.'

As it turned out, I did manage to get a lift to see Vessey after all, because much to my delight, Harriet telephoned me during the afternoon to tell me that she had come home from university and wondered if I wanted her to meet me after work. I wasn't expecting her back for another two days so I was delighted to hear from her and couldn't wait to see Ellie May turn up at the practice.

Harriet seemed as pleased to see me as I was to see her and ran straight into my arms. We kissed and I felt overjoyed that she had come into my life. 'I've missed you,' I said with deep feeling. 'I wasn't expecting you back yet.'

'I know but as I'm just revising I thought I might as well do it at home. Are you still working?'

'No, the last patient has just left. Would you mind awfully giving me a lift to Kittlewake Garage? I'm looking for a new car because the insurance company is writing mine off. Then we'll call in somewhere for a bite to eat.'

'That sounds a good idea,' said Harriet enthusiastically, 'I haven't eaten all day.'

'You shouldn't miss meals, you know; it's not good for you.'

'You're not going to start telling me off, are you, Justin? I get enough of that from my mother.'

'I'm not telling you off – I'm just concerned about you that's all.' I put my arm around her and she responded with another sensational smile.

Harriet knew where Kittlewake Garage was situated and didn't need any help to locate it but in any case, as long as you were on the right road you couldn't possibly miss it because, as Ephraim had said, there were cars everywhere stretching along the side of the road opposite the garage for at least a hundred yards in both directions. The garage itself was quite small and situated on a narrow country road where it was surrounded by fields with only a couple of houses in the vicinity. When you looked over the hedges you expected to see cattle or sheep, but instead, there were just cars. Some of them were no longer roadworthy and were used as stores for parts and equipment. It was impossible to drive on to the forecourt because there was no space that wasn't occupied by something with four wheels. The range of vehicles was enormous; most were small, relatively cheap runabouts but mixed in amongst them were some quality cars.

We had to park some distance away and as soon as we reached the premises we were approached by a slightly built, dark haired young man who sprinted athletically between the vehicles to greet us.

'I'm looking for Vessey,' I announced. 'Ephraim Trivett suggested I came to see him.'

'I'm Vessey,' he replied. 'Is Ephraim a friend of yours?'

'He's my landlord.'

'Oh I see. Are you the dentist chap?'

'Yes that's right, Justin Derwent.'

'Ephraim told me all about you yesterday. I understand you took out his tooth.'

'Yes I did, what did he tell you about me?'

'Well it was more about his tooth really. He said he couldn't understand anybody being scared of going to the dentist. He said there was absolutely nothing to it and that he didn't feel a thing and didn't even know you'd taken the tooth out. He said he'd never be scared again if he needed to have any treatment.'

'Did he really?' Patient confidentiality prevented me from saying that he was completely unaware that I had taken out his tooth because he was virtually unconscious after mixing whisky and tranquillizers.

'I'm looking for a car. Unfortunately I wrote off my last one so I need a replacement.'

'What did you have in mind? We've got all sorts here.'

'Yes I can see that. I'm not sure really. I had an Austin Healey Sprite which I liked but it was a bit cramped. I'm wondering if I might prefer something a bit bigger and more comfortable but I'd still want it to be quite nippy.'

'Let me think,' Vessey answered and his eyes scanned his stock of vehicles. 'I think I've got just the thing for you – it's that Opel Ascona over there – 1.9 litres, one owner, low mileage, in immaculate condition and quite sporty.'

'The orange one?'

'Yes, it's a smart colour don't you think?'

'They'll certainly see you coming in that,' Harriet interjected.

'Don't you like it?'

'I don't dislike it,' she added, 'it's just a bit bright but if it's a good car the colour's not that important.'

'It is a good car,' confirmed Vessey. 'I know its history and it's been well looked after. Would you like a test drive?'

'I would,' I replied, 'but I imagine it will be quite a job to get it onto the road as it's right at the back of the garage. I can come back; perhaps tomorrow.'

'You don't need to come back, I'll get it out for you; it's not a problem,' said Vessey with great positivity.

'Are you sure?'

'Absolutely,' he declared and without further ado ran off and began moving cars. All but the ones adjacent to the road had the keys in them, after all they couldn't be driven anywhere without moving the ones at the front first so there was no fear of theft. In a remarkably short time Vessey had shuffled some five cars around and the Opel was ready to be test driven on the road. 'There you go,' he announced. 'Enjoy your drive but try to be back before half past six as I've promised to take the missus out tonight.'

I looked at my watch. 'But it's only quarter past five,' I remarked.

'I know but you'll want to put it through its paces. I want you to give it a proper test run so that you're sure before you commit yourself.' He handed the keys to me.

'Don't you want to come with me?'

'No, you take the young lady for a nice drive and as long as you're back before half past six you can go where you like. There's plenty of petrol in it.'

The seats and interior were black and in perfect condition, in fact, the car looked like new. As soon as we took off I knew I was going to be impressed by it. It was smooth, quiet, comfortable and surprisingly quick on the acceleration.

'It feels nice,' remarked Harriet. 'Do you like it?'

'Yes I do. It's much more comfortable than my sports car and it's got a back seat.'

'Why exactly do you need a back seat when there's only one of you?' replied Harriet with a glint in her eye.

'To carry passengers, of course. What else? It has a radio too and a tape player.'

'I've not seen a tape player like this one before. It doesn't take the usual cassettes,' she observed, 'there's one here and it's much bigger.'

'It looks like an eight track cartridge. Put the tape in and let's see if it works.'

A few seconds later we were listening to *Sally Free and Easy* by Pentangle in high quality stereophonic sound. 'It sounds good,' I commented.

Harriet appeared less enthusiastic about it. 'The sound's all right but I don't much like the song. Unfortunately there aren't any other tapes.'

After about fifteen minutes I headed back to the garage. It was very trusting of Vessey to let me take the car out without him and I didn't think it was fair to use too much of his petrol. I had driven it far enough to know that I liked it and now it was just a question as to whether or not I could afford it.

'£1,900 is the price,' said Vessey casually, as if it were a paltry sum and not worth worrying about. As I wasn't yet sure how much the insurance company would be willing to pay for my written off sports car it was difficult to assess my ability to cover the cost of the tantalising orange beauty standing temptingly beside me.

'What do you think, Harriet?' I asked her, partly to play for more time to think and also because I hoped she would be spending some time travelling in it with me, so her opinion mattered to me.

'It isn't anything to do with me, Justin, you must do what you think is right.'

'I don't think she was very impressed with the music on the tape player,' I said to Vessey, still playing for time.

'Ah, yes the eight track cartridge player. You don't see many of those – the system never really took off; people seemed to prefer cassettes.' He was sensing my hesitation in committing myself to buy the car and decided to increase the pressure. 'I'll tell you what I'll do: I'll tax the car for a year and I'll replace the cartridge player with a cassette player.'

I looked at Harriet but she still wasn't giving away how she felt about the deal. She was making it clear that the decision had to be mine. 'All right, Vessey, you've got a deal.' I declared finally.

'I don't think you'll regret it, Justin,' he responded. 'It's a very nice car in lovely condition. When do you want to take possession of it?'

Now that I had made the decision, Harriet suddenly looked pleased for me.

'I'll give you a ring in a day or two when I've arranged the insurance and sorted out my finances,' I said to Vessey and I pulled out my cheques book. 'How much would you like me to put down as a deposit?'

'Oh don't worry about that,' said Vessey. 'Your word's good enough for me. I'll wait to hear from you.'

I thanked him and we shook hands.

'You made up your mind very quickly, Justin,' Harriet remarked as soon as we were back in Ellie May. 'I thought most men took ages when choosing a car and wouldn't make a decision until they'd been to every garage for miles around. Are you always this decisive?'

'I'm not renowned for it,' I admitted, 'in fact I'm usually quite the opposite. Do you think I've made the wrong decision?'

'No, I don't think so. It seems like a good car and I'm sure you can rely on Vessey. He's got an excellent reputation and I'm sure that if there are any problems he'll sort them out for you.'

I was about to agree with her when she brought Ellie May to a sudden stop. 'There's a baby rabbit on the side of the road and I think it's injured,' she called out. Quick as a flash she jumped out of the car and snatched up the rabbit into her arms. 'We can't leave it here, Justin, it's likely to get run over. You drive and we'll take it home with us.'

Harriet wasn't wearing her glasses but she had spotted the rabbit immediately so her eyesight couldn't be too bad. I liked to think that my eyesight was pretty good but I hadn't seen it at all. She cradled it gently on her lap and I took the wheel of Ellie May. 'Poor little thing,' she sighed, 'it's only a baby. We couldn't leave him there could we, Justin.'

'Can you tell if it's badly injured?'

'I think his back legs are broken but he doesn't seem to be in too much pain; he's lying here quietly. Let's take him back to your cottage and put him in a box with some straw where he'll feel warm and safe.'

When we got back we were able to examine its back legs and we could see they were both in a bad way. The rabbit didn't appear to be cut or bleeding but it was clear from the way its legs were hanging loosely, that they were broken.

'I don't think it will be able to recover from such injuries,' I sighed.

'Don't say that, Justin; I can't bear to see an animal suffering.'

'I know but it's badly injured.'

'So what do you suggest we do with him?'

'I don't know, Harriet. Let's make him as comfortable as possible and think about it overnight. I think we'll need to take him to a vet; Colonel Crowshaw is the local one, in fact he's the only vet I know of around here but his surgery will be closed now.'

I found a cardboard box and we asked Ephraim for some straw. He was willing enough to give us some but when he saw the rabbit he obviously didn't hold out much hope for its chances of survival.

'Doan reckon' 'ell get over that my dear,' he said to Harriet. 'Best put 'e out of 'is misery right away. I'll do it for 'ee if 'ee likes.'

'You'll do no such thing,' Harriet retorted indignantly. 'I think we should at least give him a chance.'

'Waste o' time if 'ee asks me; 'e's hurt too bad.'

Harriet lined the box with the straw and tenderly placed the little rabbit in it. 'We need to put him somewhere dark and quiet and leave him. I do hope he'll be all right, he's such a sweet little thing.' There were tears in her eyes and I put my arm around her.

'Let's go and get something to eat,' I suggested. 'We can't do any more for him now; we just need to leave him in peace.'

Harriet reluctantly agreed though I suspect she secretly wanted to keep a bedside vigil on her little patient. After a quick meal in the nearest pub, Harriet couldn't wait to get back to see if there was any change in his condition but he was still lying in the same position in his box. He looked comfortable enough though and didn't seem to be in distress.

'There's nothing we can do at the moment, Harriet. Let's have a glass of wine and relax for a while before you go home.'

Reluctantly she agreed and sat down though she was clearly very concerned about the little animal. We were chatting quietly when suddenly she spotted my old electric guitar which was half-hidden by a pile of books in the corner of the room. 'Do you play guitar?' she asked.

'I used to play in a band when I first left school but I haven't played seriously since then.'

'I bought a guitar, it's just an ordinary one, not electric but I haven't really learnt to play it – perhaps you could teach me. Will you play something for me now?'

As my playing was very rusty I was extremely reluctant. 'I haven't really played for a long time; I'm not very good now, Harriet.'

'Please, Justin; just play something I don't mind what it is.'

I picked up the guitar and switched on my little amplifier. 'I've been playing around with some Shadows tunes recently. Without backing and effects it won't sound very good but what do you think of this?'

I was about to launch into my version of *Theme for Young Lovers* which I had been practising in the evenings but then I thought that if Harriet didn't know what it was and asked me the title I might feel a bit awkward telling her. On the other hand, in view of the way I felt about her perhaps it wasn't a bad choice. I hesitated then my nerve failed me and I played a very amateurish version of *FBI* instead. I could feel the embarrassment mounting with every note due to my lack of expertise and it was a great relief when I got to the end of it.

'That's brilliant, Justin; I enjoyed it very much,' said Harriet, clapping. 'I had no idea you could play like that.'

'I need to practise more but I'd be very willing to teach you some of the basics if you'd like me to.'

'I'd like that very much. Now I'll just have a last look at the little rabbit then I must be on my way.

I didn't want her to leave but I got the impression that she was thinking that the sooner she went home, the sooner the night would pass and the sooner she could get back to her patient.

'I'll call round early tomorrow to see how he is,' said Harriet as she got into Ellie May to drive back to her parents' house.

CHAPTER THIRTY SEVEN

True to her word, Harriet was knocking on my door just after six-thirty next morning. I hadn't actually looked at the rabbit after getting out of bed; in fact I'd only been up a short time when she arrived. 'How is he?' were her first words after she had kissed me good morning.

'I haven't looked at him yet. I've not been up long and I didn't want to disturb him unnecessarily.' Without another word, Harriet went to his box and looked inside.

'He's still alive,' she pronounced with a relieved smile. 'He looks quite comfortable. Do you think we ought to give him something to eat and drink?'

'I think we should give him some water and there's some lettuce in the fridge. Try him on some of that.'

'I do hope he gets better, Justin, he's such a lovely little rabbit.'

'I hope so too, Harriet, but he is badly injured.'

'What do you think we should do with him?'

'I think we should take him to a vet. Colonel Crowshaw starts his surgery at nine o'clock, unfortunately I've got patients this morning but you could take him.'

'I wish you could come with me,' said Harriet sadly, 'but I understand that you can't, so I'll go on my own.'

Harriet drove me to my dental practice with the rabbit in his box on her back seat. 'Good luck,' I whispered and kissed her. 'Let me know how you get on.'

Spencer was in a buoyant mood when I entered the practice. 'Ah, Justin,' he called out, 'you'll be delighted to know that your new surgery is now fully operational. The engineer came yesterday, just after you left, with the parts he'd been waiting for. He's fitted them and tested everything so you're all set to go.'

'It's taken long enough,' I muttered grumpily.

'I know but surely you're pleased. I thought you couldn't wait to start using it so why are you now sounding so unenthusiastic. You're not regretting buying it are you? Is it the cost? – I know it's expensive.'

'No I don't regret buying it and I am pleased, it's just that Harriet and I found an injured rabbit yesterday and we're both upset because it's in a bad way – I don't think it's going to survive. She's taking it to the vet's this morning.'

'It's obvious you aren't a countryman, Justin, if you were you wouldn't be getting all emotional about a rabbit; there are thousands of them out there. Most country folk think the best place for rabbits is in a stew and the farmers would like to get rid of them completely because they see them as pests.'

'Well we think differently and what you say doesn't apply to all country folk because Harriet was born and brought up in the country.'

'Harriet? Is she your latest conquest?' Spencer enquired with a glint in his eye.

'I wouldn't describe her as a *conquest*. She's just a friend.'

'So is it serious?' he persisted.

He seized upon my hesitation in answering and his face broke into a broad grin. 'It is, isn't it? My goodness.' Then somewhat unkindly, I thought, he remarked, 'let's hope you have more luck with this one than you did with the last two.'

I decided that his statement wasn't worthy of a comment and I started to move off to go and look at my new surgery. "Before you go, Justin, there's something else I wanted to talk to you about. Have you heard of Toothplan?'

'No I can't say I have. What is it?'

'It's really exciting. It's a scheme for providing patients with private treatment – an alternative to the National Health. We're always saying we'd like to do more private treatment and not have to suffer the constraints of the health service and this is a way we can do it. Patients who sign up to the scheme pay us a regular monthly amount by direct debit and in return for this we provide them with all the treatment they need. Once they're signed up there's no more paperwork, no prior approvals, and if they don't turn up we still get paid and we also get paid whilst we're on holiday because the direct debits continue. At the moment, we've no idea how much we'll earn over the next few months because we don't know how many patients will be coming in for treatment and if none of them come, we don't earn a penny. Under this scheme, we know that the direct debits will be paid into our bank and so it removes a lot of the uncertainty. Don't you think it sounds a great scheme?'

'On the face of it but I can think of a lot of questions I'd like answers to before I can really say whether I think it's a good scheme or not.'

'Well of course, Justin, but I understand there are a lot of practices up and down the country that are going over to it and with considerable success. For the scheme to work you've obviously got to sell the idea to your patients and get them to sign up. I can see that some dentists, you included possibly, might find this difficult because salesmanship is not something dentists are trained in though I don't think that I, personally, would have too much trouble. Anyway, there's a course in Dorchester on the fifth of next month and I've signed us up for it. It's an all-day course designed to explain fully how the scheme operates. You'll have a chance to ask questions about it and there are also practical instructions on how to go about selling the idea to patients. I'm really looking forward to it. I've told Beryl to cross out the day in my appointment book and you need to get Wendy to do the same with yours.'

I wondered if this would turn out to be another of Spencer's innovative ideas that proved to be a complete waste of time and energy. Perhaps I wasn't in the mood to consider such a radical change in the way we operated our practice because I was too preoccupied with the rabbit and my new surgery at this very moment. However, he seemed fairly insistent that I should at least give the matter some serious consideration and I was prepared to do so but not right now.

I was very anxious to start using my new surgery but I really needed a bit of time to get to know the equipment and practise with it before treating patients. I had a busy morning ahead of me and I decided that it might be best to continue in my old surgery today and then spend some time at the end of the afternoon familiarising myself with the new set up so that I could start in earnest tomorrow. Spencer looked aghast when I told him that this was my plan.

'I'm sorry, Justin, but I thought you'd want to get in there immediately. I'm afraid I've already started dismantling your old surgery because I've got plans for that room; you'll have to use your new one.'

'Thanks, Spencer,' I grunted sarcastically. At that moment Wendy arrived. 'It seems we're in here, Wendy. Spencer couldn't wait to throw us out from our room upstairs.'

'That's good, Justin,' she exclaimed, you must be delighted that your new surgery is ready at last. There seem to have been so many delays in getting all the parts for it. Are all the hand instruments still upstairs, Spencer?'

'Err, no,' Spencer replied shiftily. 'I emptied all the drawers and put everything in boxes which are on the worktop in the new surgery.'

'Oh my goodness,' exclaimed Wendy, 'I wish you'd told me. It's going to take ages to sort them all out and the first patient's due in a few minutes.'

Spencer slunk away without another word but he looked guilty that he had created a difficult situation for Wendy and me. I wondered why on earth he was in such a hurry to push me out of my upstairs surgery. He obviously had plans for the room which he hadn't yet divulged to me.

Fortunately, my first three patients of the morning were all for routine check-ups which gave Wendy an opportunity to begin organizing the instruments and pack them away neatly in the new cabinets. It was quite a big job and I had hoped that we would have the chance to do it in a more leisurely and ordered way but Spencer had dashed all hope of that. I had been looking forward to starting work in my new surgery for several weeks now but I would have preferred to have eased myself into it a bit more gently than this.

I kept wondering how Harriet was getting on at the vet's. She was hoping to catch Colonel Crowshaw before he started his surgery and I wondered how she would accept it if he told her that he couldn't help the little rabbit. I didn't have to wait long to find out and the fact that tears were streaming down her face told me it had not been good news.

'The vet's put him down,' she sobbed. 'He said the back legs were so badly broken they wouldn't have healed and a rabbit with no back legs wouldn't be able to survive. He also said that he would have

246

been in a lot of pain even though he didn't appear to be, so the kindest thing was to put him to sleep.'

'I'm so sorry, Harriet,' I said, putting my arm around her.

'I didn't want the vet to dispose of him so I asked if I could have him back. Can we bury him when you've finished work?'

'Yes, of course.' I was touched by her sensitivity and the amount of compassion she showed for the little animal and it endeared me to her even more. I hoped that the grief she was feeling would soon pass and that she would not get too depressed. 'Try not to be too upset; perhaps he's gone to a better place,' I said comfortingly. 'What are you going to do for the rest of the day?'

'I'm going to the library to do some revision.'

'Shall I meet you at lunchtime?'

'Yes, I'd like that,' she replied. 'I'll come to the surgery and pick you up.'

I watched her walk down the path and get into her car and once again the realization hit me that I had never felt the same way about anyone else before. It was becoming very serious as far as I was concerned and whilst I was fairly certain she liked me I wasn't at all sure if there was any real depth to her feelings. I waited until she had driven off and reflected on just how much I was looking forward to seeing her again at lunchtime. In the meantime, I had the challenge of a complete new surgery to contend with.

Although my new equipment was very different from that which Spencer had provided for me, it was actually quite similar to what I had been used to at dental school and after an hour I was already beginning to feel at home with it. After two hours, I was positively enjoying using it. Everything fell conveniently to hand and made the practice of dentistry much more effortless. I really felt that it would make my life a lot easier and I would be able to undertake more ambitious procedures such as multiple crowns and extensive bridges. This would be good for the practice and also, hopefully, for my bank balance. At eleven o'clock, Mr Dransfield was booked in to have a back tooth prepared for a crown and when I started the morning I was very apprehensive about having to do this in a strange surgery but by the time eleven o'clock arrived I was perfectly relaxed about it; in fact, I was looking forward to it.

'It's a fabulous surgery,' remarked Wendy who had considerable experience of working in many dental practices both old and new and she was quite clearly enjoying working in the new surroundings. Her professionalism prevented her from being too critical of Spencer's ancient equipment but I knew that she was amazed just how primitive it was compared with most other dental practices.

'This is rather smart,' remarked Mr Dransfield, as Wendy ushered him into my new workplace. 'It's a great improvement on your surgery upstairs; I would say that you've left the last century behind you and moved up to date.'

'I'm glad you like it, Mr Dransfield. Please take a seat. We only started using it this morning but already it feels really good.'

'I expect you'll be charging me twice as much for my treatment now to pay for all this,' he joked.

'I promise you my fees haven't gone up. I'm hoping that the new equipment will make me more efficient so the surgery will eventually pay for itself.'

'I'll bet that's what the sales rep told you,' he replied with a cynical grin. 'Anyway I hope it proves to be the case.'

Mr Dransfield was no lightweight and I watched with consternation as he dumped himself on to my green faux leather upholstery with about as much grace as a sack of potatoes with scant regard for the fact that my chair was less than two hours into its working life. I suppressed my desire to pass comment and Wendy handed me a syringe so that I could administer local anaesthetic.

After waiting a few minutes for the injection to take effect I reached for my shiny new high speed handpiece and began to prepare Mr Dransfield's tooth. The drilling was smooth and effortless and I was amazed how quickly and effectively it removed tooth substance. I had almost completed the preparation when quite unexpectedly everything came to a stop. The operating light and the lights in the surgery all went out and I realised that there must be a power cut. 'How annoying,' I exclaimed. 'I'm sorry, Mr Dransfield, I don't know what the problem is but the electricity has gone off; hopefully it will come back on again soon. In the meantime I suggest we just hang on and see what happens. Wendy went to check that the power loss was affecting the whole practice and not just my surgery and came back to confirm that Spencer was without electricity also and the waiting room was plunged into darkness. Whilst we were waiting to see if the situation changed, Spencer's next patient arrived and was able to inform us that there had been an accident just down the road and that a car had collided with an electricity link box. This was undoubtedly the reason for the power loss. I had no idea how long it was likely to be before I could work again and after fifteen minutes I decided I would have to postpone Mr Dransfield's treatment to another day. I dressed his tooth as best I could in the available light and asked Wendy to arrange another appointment for him.

As Mr Dransfield stood up I was horrified to see a large bunch of keys hanging out of his back pocket. Whilst sitting on them must have been uncomfortable, my greater concern was for my new chair which had a large indentation corresponding to the point of contact between the seat and the keys, but worse still, there was a definite tear in the upholstery about an inch long. I was mortified to the point where I couldn't really believe what my eyes were seeing. My fingers explored the defect to provide a second opinion and tragically reached the same conclusion – the keys had cut the leather. It wouldn't have mattered so much had I still been using the old chair upstairs but for it to happen to my brand new one, on the very first morning, was hard to bear. It had cost me a fortune; or rather it would do eventually as I hadn't even started paying for it yet. Mr Dransfield saw me looking at the damage but he said nothing and his expression did not disclose whether or not he knew what he'd done.

I shuffled off to Spencer's surgery just in time to see him transporting the ancient foot treadle drill into his surgery. It was quite a while since he had last used it and it had been lying around in a cupboard, consequently, dust was lying thickly over the rust and flaking black paint. Strapped to his head was a lamp very much like coal miners wear on their helmets.

'The electricity could be off for some time,' he called out. 'Last time that link box was damaged we were without power for seven hours. That's why I've made contingency arrangements. With this headlight and foot drill I can carry on working without mains electricity.'

'What about your chair? Don't you need power to make that go up and down?'

'Works off compressed air and there'll be enough in the tank to keep me going for a long time. It's the only surviving compressed air operated chair in the entire country according to the dental supply company's engineer.'

He sounded quite proud of the fact that he owned what was probably the most outdated dental chair in existence.

'You're not really going to drill some poor blighter's tooth with that contraption, are you?' I asked, looking at the primitive piece of equipment he was carrying.

'I certainly am,' he confirmed. 'Time's money and we can't afford to sit around twiddling our thumbs. So much for your fancy new equipment,' he scoffed, 'without electricity it's useless.'

'Mr Dransfield has just ripped my chair,' I announced glumly. 'He had a bunch of keys in his back pocket.'

'On the first morning!' he shrieked. Although his shocked response had a note of sympathy I thought I detected a hint of a grin on his face as he said it. 'The stuff they cover the chairs with these days is rubbish – it won't last five minutes. The upholstery on mine is still as good as the day it was made.'

CHAPTER THIRTY EIGHT

I had arranged insurance cover for the car I was buying from Vessey at Kittlewake Garage and much to my amazement the insurance company had paid what I thought was a very fair sum for my written-off sports car. I had contacted my bank and explained the circumstances and they had readily agreed to give me a loan to cover the balance so I was all set to collect my new car and was intending to pick it up later that day. I should have been happy but something else was causing me concern. For some days now I had been experiencing chest pain. At first I didn't pay much attention to it and I thought it would go away but it didn't. It wasn't severe but it did seem to be slowly getting worse and I couldn't help wondering if it was the onset of heart trouble. It seemed unlikely at my age but it wasn't unheard of for young people to have heart attacks and my imagination was starting to go into overdrive. I had some medical knowledge so I ought to be able to make a sensible diagnosis but for some reason, when it concerns oneself, common sense seems to go out of the window. I tried analysing the pain: it wasn't intense and it didn't radiate to my arms. Strenuous exercise didn't seem to make it worse so I should have concluded that it probably wasn't heart pain but I found it difficult to reach a rational conclusion.

Harriet had sensed that something was troubling me and although I denied it to start with, I finally shared my anxiety with her.

'I shouldn't think there's anything wrong with your heart; it's most unlikely at your age,' she stated reassuringly, 'but the best way to put your mind at rest is to make an appointment to see the doctor and get it checked out.'

'I'm not sure if I've got a doctor now. Mine died at the wheel of his car – of a heart attack as a matter of fact.'

'How old was he?' Harriet enquired.

'Sixty something.'

'Considerably older than you, then. Be sensible, Justin. How many men of your age do you hear about dying of heart attacks?'

'It does happen occasionally.'

'Yes but it's extremely unusual and I can't believe there's anything wrong with your heart – you look well enough to me. As I said, the best thing you can do is go and phone the doctor right away; there must be a doctor standing in at the practice even if he's not there permanently.'

'I hate seeing doctors. Perhaps I'll wait another day or two to see if the pain gets better.'

'I think you should go and get checked out immediately then at least you'll know one way or the other. Do you want me to phone up and make an appointment for you?'

'Would you mind?'

Without further ado, Harriet phoned Dr MacKean's surgery. I heard her say, 'yes that will be fine, thank you very much.' She turned to me. 'They'll see you at four fifteen.'

'Today?'

'Of course, today. It's important to get this sorted as soon as possible. We can pick up your new car up immediately afterwards.'

'Unless I'm sent to hospital,' I commented half-jokingly.

'Don't be ridiculous,' Harriet scoffed. 'I don't think there's anything wrong with you; I only suggested going to see the doctor to put your mind at rest.'

When four fifteen arrived we were sitting in the doctor's waiting room. The last time I was there was when I went to see Dr MacKean for my insurance medical. That wasn't a particularly pleasant experience either but Dr MacKean hadn't found anything wrong with my heart then and it wasn't that long ago so perhaps Harriet was right – I was making a fuss about nothing and there wasn't anything wrong with me.

The room was much more attractive now compared with the last time I saw it. The walls had been painted a fresh, pale blue and the tattered old curtains had been replaced with new ones. The dingy old prints which were dismal and depressing had been replaced with vibrant images of racing cars and there was an interesting variety of new magazines on the low table in the middle of the room. They confirmed that someone at the practice was keen on motor sport and I was surprised to see amongst them a music magazine with a picture of a Gibson guitar on the front cover. Harriet spotted it as well. 'It looks as if someone else is interested in guitars; it might be the new doctor. If so, you should ask him about it; perhaps you could do some playing together.'

'I don't know about that; I'm not good enough to be thinking about playing with someone else – he might be brilliant.'

'Nonsense, Justin; I thought you were very good.'

'It's nice of you to say so, Harriet but I'm under no illusions about my guitar playing ability. I'm happy just to play on my own for my personal enjoyment.'

Looking around the waiting room it did look as if someone had taken over on a permanent basis. I thought it unlikely that someone filling the post temporarily would have implemented these changes.

At two minutes after four fifteen a door opened and a cheerful young man emerged from what I knew to be the consulting room. He was of medium height and build with a mop of dark brown hair and a beard. His eyes twinkled through gold rimmed spectacles and he held out his hand to shake mine.

'Dermot Fitzpatrick,' he announced, 'you must be Justin Derwent.' His accent was unmistakeably southern Irish and its soft, almost musical quality together with his relaxed manner was instantly soothing. He had a confident and reassuring air about him and his very presence immediately made me feel less anxious.

'You work with Spencer Padginton, don't you?' he continued. 'We have many mutual patients and I have to say that although I've only been here a short time I've heard some very complimentary remarks about your dental practice.'

'That's nice to know. We do our best to keep the patients happy but it isn't always easy. Nobody likes going to the dentist.'

'You're dead right,' he agreed. 'Though it's not really surprising, because after all, you chaps do inflict pain.'

'We try hard not to but dental treatment can be uncomfortable.'

'You can say that again. Speaking of which, I really must come and get my teeth sorted out; I keep spitting out broken pieces and whilst I'm not getting any pain at the moment, I ought to get them looked at.'

When he smiled he displayed a set of very strong-looking, even white teeth which showed absolutely no sign of the mishaps he was referring to.

'Have you taken over the practice from Dr MacKean permanently?'

'Yes, I'm originally from Dublin and I've been working in orthopaedics at Poole Hospital for the past two years but I always intended going into general practice and I was looking for a small country practice. I think this will suit me fine. We, that's my wife and I, are already feeling settled here and we love it.' He looked at Harriet. 'Is this your lovely wife?'

'No, we aren't married,' I replied. I was about to say that we were just friends but I stopped myself because I suppose I didn't want to convey to Harriet that was how I saw her. 'This is Harriet and it was she who decided I ought to come and see you to get checked out. If it hadn't been for her I probably wouldn't be here now.'

'Hello, Harriet,' he said warmly as he shook hands with her. 'I hate to admit it but it's often the case that it's the women in our lives who help us to see sense. Do you find that being unmarried is a disadvantage in your job as a dentist? It would be a disadvantage for me as a doctor.'

'I think it's a bit different.'

'You're probably right,' he agreed. 'Anyway come through to the surgery.'

He remained silent and attentive whilst I described my symptoms in detail.

'It's most unlikely that you've got heart trouble,' he exclaimed. 'You don't smoke, you aren't overweight and the pain doesn't seem to be linked to exercise.' He pulled out his stethoscope. 'Unbutton your shirt and let's have a listen.'

His examination was brief but he seemed happy with what he heard. 'You've got a heart like a jungle drum, Justin. Without an ECG and more tests I can't be absolutely certain but I'm more than ninety-five percent sure your heart's fine.'

'I feel a bit stupid now; I should have known that the symptoms didn't point to heart trouble.'

'Don't feel stupid; it's always difficult to make an accurate diagnosis on yourself or even members of your family.'

'So what do you think is causing the pain?'

'Could be several things but not likely to be anything to worry about. If pressed I would say that you might have a touch of oesophagitis which will probably get better in a few days. Perhaps you should add a little water to your whisky instead of taking it neat or stick to beer like I do. It could also be caused through not eating sensibly which tends to be very common amongst single young men; what you need is a wife to look after you. Have you and Harriet got plans?'

'I haven't known her very long.' I paused before adding, 'but who knows?'

He smiled. 'I don't think there's any need to give you a prescription; as I said it will probably clear up in a day or two. If it doesn't come and see me again.'

'Thanks, doctor; you've put my mind at rest.'

'Call me Dermot. Now on a more important note, on Thursday evenings I and a number of other doctors and young professional people go to a little pub called the Sportsman out towards Chiselton. Do you know it?'

'No, I don't think I do.'

'It's a bit rough but there's a great atmosphere and it gives those of us who are married a chance to get away from the family for an hour or two. They're a very friendly bunch of people and it would be really good if you were to join us; we haven't got any general dental practitioners so far, though there is an orthodontist. Would you like to come?'

'Yes I would, very much. Thanks for the invitation.'

'Okay, I'll pick you up at six o'clock; I've got your address on your record card. I, and two other doctors who live locally, take turns to drive and unfortunately it's my turn this week so sadly I shall be on orange juice but if you join the rota it will mean that each of us only has to drive every fourth week, though that isn't the reason I've invited you – well not entirely. We start about six o'clock and I'm usually back home by nine, though we have been known to be quite a bit later, but that's only when I'm not driving.' He grinned as he said it and I could see that he was someone who enjoyed social gatherings and, in true Irish tradition, was probably very fond of a drink or two. I wanted to make new friends and it seemed to me that this would be an excellent opportunity which I was very pleased to seize.

'I shall look forward to that, thank you.'

Harriet looked apprehensive as I re-entered the waiting room but my relieved expression immediately convinced her that Dermot had been able to allay my fears. Before I had time to give her any information she blurted out, 'I told you that you didn't have heart trouble. So what is wrong with you, if anything?'

'He thinks I might have oesophagitis but it should go away in a few days. He says I need someone to look after me because I'm probably not eating properly. In fact, I feel better already.'

'It's amazing what a bit of reassurance can do,' she ribbed, as she squeezed my arm and treated me to another winning smile. 'Come on, let's go and collect your new car then, when we get back, I'll make sure you get a good meal.'

The orange Opel was the first car I saw as we approached Vessey's garage. Its gleaming paintwork was almost dazzling and left me in no doubt that Vessey had spent time polishing it in anticipation of my arrival. I was pleased to see that it was standing at the very front of the huge assortment of vehicles and positioned so that it could be driven away immediately without any need for intricate manoeuvring. As I stood admiring it, Vessey appeared from nowhere. 'She looks good, doesn't she?' he called out.

I think he was referring to the car but as he was looking at Harriet as he said it, I wasn't exactly sure. However, I couldn't disagree with him either way.

'I'm afraid I have a confession to make,' he continued. 'I clean forgot about changing the tape player. I'm really sorry but it just went completely out of my head. I will do it for you, of course, but you'll need to come back. I only remembered about it just before you arrived. I'm really sorry.'

'That's all right, Vessey. I can come back when it's convenient for you – I really don't mind.'

'Does that mean I have to go on listening to *Sally Free and Easy* for a while longer?' Harriet asked with a smile.

'I promise I won't switch it on if you really can't stand it,' I replied, feeling pleased that she was obviously willing to go on being my companion.

CHAPTER THIRTY NINE

The next morning I told Spencer that I had met the new doctor who had taken over Dr MacKean's practice. Spencer wasn't a bit interested in why I had been to see him and showed no concern whatsoever for my state of health.

'Did you ask him if he's willing to give dental anaesthetics so we can resume our GA sessions?' were his first words.

'No I didn't, Spencer – you know my views on that. You'll have to ask him yourself – I'm having nothing to do with it.'

'Did he say that he'd had anything to do with anaesthetics in the past or give any indication that he might be willing to help us out.'

'No he didn't. He's young and has been working in orthopaedics at Poole hospital for the past two years so I think it's unlikely he's had anything to do with dental anaesthesia.'

'Pity,' Spencer mumbled looking slightly crestfallen. 'Anyway, I still think it might be worth asking him. You never know, he might be willing to do a bit of extra training to extend his skills. I'll probably phone him up quite soon and sound him out. I don't suppose you'll be seeing him again in the near future?'

'As a matter of fact, I'm going out for a drink with him and some other GPs on Thursday but I'm not going to mention it; you'll have to speak to him yourself.'

'Other GPs! Well there must be one of them prepared to do a bit of gassing for us. You've got a golden opportunity to help move our practice forward, Justin. You must speak to them about it.'

'I'm sorry, Spencer, but I've told you; I want nothing to do with GA ever again.'

'I'm amazed by your attitude, Justin, I'm constantly being asked by patients if they can have gas and I feel I'm letting them down when I tell them we don't do it here. I also think we're missing a valuable opportunity to expand our practice and I'm convinced it could prove highly lucrative.'

'The previous attempt wasn't very lucrative, as I recall. In fact, the session finished up costing you twenty-five guineas, not to mention the time we both wasted.'

'That was unfortunate and it was because we didn't really have enough time to arrange the session properly. It will be different next time.'

'As far as I'm concerned there won't be a next time. None of my patients has ever asked me for gas so I'm very surprised when you say that you are constantly being asked. If anyone does want or need GA then I shall refer them to hospital.'

'Ah well, that doesn't entirely get them off your hands.'

'What do you mean?'

'This very afternoon I'm going along to the oral surgery department of Dorchester hospital to remove Mr Dickson's upper eight. He's one of the patients who has insisted that he must have a GA for his extraction. As we can't do it here at present, I referred him to the hospital and they wrote back saying that they'll provide the theatre, the nursing staff and the anaesthetist but I must go along to carry out the extraction.'

'That's a bit much, Spencer. They've got enough staff there; surely one of them could carry out a simple extraction without you having to give up an entire afternoon and go all the way there to do their job for them.'

'Actually, I'm quite looking forward to it as it will give me an opportunity to show the people who work at the hospital just how skilful and efficient we are at removing teeth. I sometimes think that they look upon us general practitioners as the poor relations. I don't mean "poor" financially – in fact they think we're overpaid; I mean "poor" in that we aren't as clever as those who work in the hospital. But you're right when you say I have to give up what would have been my afternoon off and of course, I shan't get paid for it which is why I say it would be a good thing if we could offer GA here.'

Spencer looked very smart as he got into his Rolls Royce to drive to the hospital. He hated wearing a suit normally but this was one of those occasions when he felt it was necessary. He chose a dark grey pinstripe with matching waistcoat complete with gold watch chain and he carried a well-worn leather Gladstone bag though I don't think there was actually anything in it because the hospital would provide the necessary instruments but it was all part of the overall image that Spencer wished to convey.

He arrived at the hospital with plenty of time to spare before the 'operation' was due to take place. Having parked his car with great precision in one of the bays reserved for hospital staff, he swaggered to reception and asked for directions to the oral surgery department. He strutted through the maze of corridors following the blue and white signs and was greeted by a nurse who told him where he could change his outdoor clothing for surgical attire before scrubbing up and putting on a gown and surgical gloves. He knew he could not go into the operating theatre wearing his shoes so he selected a pair of white rubber boots from the row in the corner of the room. The fact that they were clearly marked with the name 'Professor Charles Humbert-Prestwich didn't worry him in the slightest – they were the right size and that was all that mattered. After all he was only borrowing them for a short time and as Professor Humbert-Prestwich was an eminent surgeon, he couldn't think of anyone else whose shoes he would prefer to step into to.

He was meticulous about scrubbing his arms and hands with antiseptic soap and refused to be rushed into skimping the procedure. It may only have been a tooth extraction but Spencer was out to show that he attached considerable importance to the high standards of sterility expected of all surgeons carrying out operations. It made no difference whether it was major heart surgery or a simple dental extraction, the same level of infection control had to be adopted. A nurse helped him on with his green gown and gloves and he made his entrance into the operating theatre where Mr Dickson was already on the operating table receiving the attention of the anaesthetist. Many general practitioners would have felt a little bit apprehensive in that sort of situation as it was not something they experienced very often, if ever, but Spencer was perfectly relaxed about the whole thing. 'Good afternoon, everyone,' he announced.

He waited patiently whilst the anaesthetist satisfied himself that the patient was unconscious and that his throat had been closed off to prevent anything accidentally slipping down it. Finally, the anaesthetist invited Spencer to proceed. 'He's all yours Mr Padginton.'

'Thank you,' Spencer replied and stepped forward. 'A mouth mirror, if you will, please nurse,' he demanded, holding out his hand. 'Will you please adjust the light –that's perfect – thank you very much.'

'What forceps do you want?' asked the nurse in a tone which suggested that it was somewhat beneath her to be assisting with such a mundane procedure when she was used to being involved in much more complicated operations.

'I shall need a straight Warwick James to elevate the tooth from its socket and a pair of 101 forceps to deliver it,' replied Spencer, determined to demonstrate that although the nurse might think that extracting a tooth was simple, he would nevertheless accomplish it with considerable panache.

The instruments were duly presented to Spencer and in a matter of seconds the offending tooth clattered satisfyingly into the kidney bowl held by the nurse just inches away from the patient's mouth. 'That's it,' Spencer declared, 'please insert a gauze pack, nurse, and thank you all very much for your assistance. I wish you good day.'

With that he left the theatre and returned Professor Humbert-Prestwich's boots to their original position. When he got back to the practice he couldn't wait to speak to me.

'How did it go, Spencer?' I enquired.

'Oh fine, Justin, the extraction was no problem at all. I think the hospital staff were quite amazed at the speed and efficiency with which I carried out the procedure. Of course, in general practice, time's money so we are used to working quickly, whilst at the hospital, they can take as long as they like and because of this, they are actually very slow workers. I think it came as a bit of a surprise to them to see me extract the tooth in a flash. But I have to say that I was extremely impressed by the sheer cleanliness and sterility of the set-up at the hospital. Whilst driving back I found myself wondering if our cross-infection control might be a bit lacking.'

'We sterilise our instruments and the nurses wipe down the surfaces between patients; what more should we do?'

'There's a lot we could do. For example, I don't think it's acceptable just to put on a white coat on top of our outdoor clothes. We really ought to strip right off and wear something completely different in the surgery and if there's any suggestion at all of it becoming contaminated we should change completely. I also think we should be wearing hats, face masks and gloves when we're operating.'

'I'd feel a bit foolish wearing all that just to treat people's teeth. In fact, I think it might put some of them off; particularly children. There's no evidence that patients are getting infections or suffering harm due to the way we work and we're following current guidelines for cross-infection control. You're not suggesting we throw away our hot-air and boiling water sterilisers and get an autoclave are you, Spencer?'

He hesitated. 'You should see the autoclaves they have at the hospital – they're fantastic and obviously sterilise instruments much more effectively than we can with our simple equipment but all autoclaves are very expensive, even smaller ones. Perhaps it's something we could think about for the future because we do owe it to our patients to provide the best for them. We're never going to be able to match the infection control the hospital can achieve but I'm convinced we should look at our procedures and concentrate on implementing a completely aseptic technique at all times. You say that patients are not getting infections but you don't know that for certain. Take infected sockets following extractions, for example – we get quite a few of those.'

'It happens occasionally but we don't get many and I don't think it's anything to do with the way we operate; infected sockets just happen. When you think how the mouth is teaming with bacteria, I'm just amazed that more sockets don't become infected.'

'Well, seeing the way things are done at the hospital has certainly made me think. We really do need to ask ourselves if we are really doing everything possible for our patients with regards making sure they don't get unnecessary infections. Today was a real eye-opener for me. The lengths they go to at the hospital in order to ensure sterility and prevent patients becoming infected were exemplary and truly outstanding. After all, even one infected socket is one too many if it could be avoided by stricter control. I have decided to incorporate some of their methods into this practice so over the next few days I shall be drawing up details of a new regime we must adopt for the future.

CHAPTER FORTY

I was looking forward to an evening at home alone. The only person I would have been pleased to see was Harriet and she was away at university so I intended to use the time to catch up with some paperwork and maybe go for a walk later on. I was about to sit down to a sandwich and a cup of tea when the telephone rang.

'Hello, Justin, it's Sarah Hanson here. How are you?'

I was taken by surprise when I heard her voice as I wasn't expecting it to be her on the phone. My heart sank a little. 'I'm very well thank you, Sarah. How are you?'

'I'm well, Justin. I hope you don't mind my phoning you – I wouldn't have, but my mother asked me to get in touch with you because she has a favour to ask. I said that it wasn't fair to trouble you but she doesn't have anyone else she could turn to and she said she was sure you wouldn't mind. I know that things are over between you and me and I assure you there are no strings attached.'

'I'll help if I can, Sarah. What does your mother want?'

'Well, she's decided she wants a serving hatch between the kitchen and the dining room which means knocking a hole in the wall. It's not a huge job but it's a bit more than mother and I could manage on our own and she wondered if you would be prepared to come over and give us a hand. It probably wouldn't take more than a couple of hours. I said she should employ a builder but because it's only a small job it's difficult to get one to do it. They seem to want to charge over the odds and they make such a mess. Please say if you really don't want to do it, Justin, but mother would be so grateful if you would be prepared to help. There'll be a bottle or two of wine in it for you.'

It was one of those situations when I wanted to be helpful but I was a bit concerned about possible repercussions. I had met Harriet now and I didn't want to rekindle any flames with respect to my relationship with Sarah, though she did say there were no strings attached. However, I certainly wouldn't have wanted Harriet to know that I was going to Sarah's house so if I did go, I would have to hide it from her but at the same time I didn't want to deceive her. It was a very awkward situation to be in.

'I'll understand if you say no, Justin,' Sarah continued, 'but my mother would be so grateful.'

'When would you want me to come?'

'Whenever it suits you.'

'Do you want me to come this evening?'

'Well, yes if you like. That would be great. I'm not going out anywhere and my mother certainly isn't. Yes it would be wonderful if you could come this evening.'

'All right, I'll just grab a bite to eat and then I'll come.'

'Why don't you come now and you can eat with us – then you won't have to bother cooking.'

'I wasn't intending to do much cooking, Sarah. I was just going to make a sandwich.'

'I've made a chicken and mushroom pie so you can come and have some of that.'

'Sounds good. All right then, I'll come straight away.'

I had very mixed feelings as I drove my new Opel to Sarah's house. I felt sorry for Sarah's mother who wasn't in the best of health and I wanted to help her but at the same time I couldn't help thinking about Harriet. I didn't feel I would be able to tell her I had been to see Sarah because I wasn't sure she would understand. On the other hand, if I didn't tell her and she happened to find out later, she would probably be very upset that I hadn't been open about it and that might make matters even worse. I came to the conclusion that, if I had been sensible, I would have made some excuse to Sarah and kept away, but it was too late for that now.

Sarah was waiting at her door as I drove up to her house. She spotted my new car immediately.

'I like your car, Justin; it's really smart,' she exclaimed, kissing me quickly on the cheek. 'Have you got rid of your sports car?'

'I'm afraid I wrote it off.'

'That's awful. Were you hurt?'

'Amazingly no I wasn't, but my car was a terrible mess.'

'That's a shame because I know you loved that car.'

'That's true I did but this is more comfortable and certainly roomier. It's actually quite sporty as well.'

'It looks lovely. Anyway come in.'

'Ah Justin, how lovely to see you again,' said her mother warmly, 'would you like a beer or a whisky?'

'A beer would be nice, thank you.'

'Get Justin a beer, please Sarah. I'm so grateful to you for offering to help with this serving hatch. I've drawn it out on the wall so you can see where it will go. It's a brick wall which is why I didn't feel Sarah and I could do it on our own but I'm sure it won't take you very long because I expect your arms are quite strong through extracting teeth. I've got a hammer and chisel which is probably all you'll need. Anyway, sit down and drink your beer and we'll eat first to build up your energy before you tackle the wall.'

The pie that Sarah had baked was absolutely delicious and having consumed two large helpings accompanied by a delightful Sauvignon Blanc followed by profiteroles with raspberries and cream I felt more like sleeping than knocking a hole in the wall. As it turned out, the job was completed very quickly with little effort as the plaster on the wall was crumbly and the bricks relatively soft.

'Don't worry about the mess, Justin, Sarah and I can clean that up later. In any case, apart from a bit of dust there isn't much. You go and sit down and I'll get you a brandy and some coffee – you've earned it.'

'Just coffee please, Mrs Hanson. I have to drive home very shortly and I don't want to write off this car like I did the last one.'

'Go into the drawing room with Sarah and I'll get the coffee.'

Suddenly I felt a bit awkward when Sarah and I were alone together. She sat down beside me on the sofa and her eyes became fixed upon mine. There was absolutely no sign of the volatile nature I had sampled the last time I went out with her when I told her we had no future together.

'Thank you so much for coming, Justin. Mother and I really appreciate your help and it's lovely to see you again. Is life treating you well?'

'Yes, thank you Sarah. How about you?' I replied, trying to shift the attention from me to her. I was hoping she wouldn't ask if there was anyone else in my life as I didn't want to talk to her about Harriet. On the other hand, I didn't want to lie by saying there wasn't anyone else especially if it encouraged her to think that there was a chance that we might get back together.

When I left to drive back home, I couldn't help wondering if the request for me to help with the serving hatch had merely been a ploy, perhaps on the part of Sarah's mother, to get Sarah and me to meet up again in the hope of some sort of reconciliation. I'm quite sure that Sarah would have had the strength to knock out a few bricks as she wasn't exactly weak physically or there must have been someone other than me they could have asked to help. I did, however, like Sarah and I didn't want to hurt her but my feelings for Harriet were taking off in a way that I had never experienced before and in a way that had not happened when I was with Sarah.

CHAPTER FORTY ONE

At five to six on Thursday evening, Dermot zoomed up to my cottage in his sleek silver Golf Gti and screeched to a halt outside my door.

'I like your car, Dermot; is it new?'

'Hi, Justin. Yes I bought it just over a month ago. I had a black one before this but my wife said it made me look like a funeral director which isn't really the right image for a GP. I doubt if anyone else thought that but I seized upon it as an excuse to justify buying a new car.'

'Was that a Golf Gti?'

'Yes I love them. They go like the clappers; in fact they are the nippiest cars on the road at the price.'

'It looks great.'

'You can drive it to the pub if you like.'

'Thanks Dermot but I'd be too worried about smashing it up.'

'I'm sure you won't do that.'

I was thankful that he didn't press the issue and I jumped into the passenger seat.

'I would normally have Chris and Alan with me but they can't come this evening. Chris is a GP and Alan is an anaesthetist and we take turns to do the driving. If you join us it will mean that I only have to drive every fourth week instead of every third, which will be great.'

When I heard the word 'anaesthetist' I was tempted for a moment to mention that Spencer was looking for someone to give gas for dental procedures but then I decided to keep quiet about it. Dermot didn't say anything so I assumed Spencer hadn't yet contacted him.

I don't think Dermot was deliberately trying to impress me with the car's performance but if he was, he certainly succeeded. We covered the eight miles to 'The Sportsman Inn' along the narrow, winding, country roads faster than I believed was possible. Although his driving was extremely fast he was completely in control throughout the journey and no time did I feel unsafe. I suddenly remembered the motor sport magazines in his waiting room and the pictures of racing cars on the walls. 'I take it you're a motor racing fan?'

'Yes very much so, I love watching it on television and I go to see it live whenever I can. I suppose you saw the pictures in my waiting room?'

'I did and the magazines. Are you interested in music as well?' I asked, thinking about the guitar magazine I'd noticed.

'I have a guitar and I used to play in a band but I haven't played much for some time.'

His words encouraged me somewhat. Perhaps he wasn't so brilliant that I would find it daunting to play with him. 'I also used to play in a band many years ago,' I replied. 'I still have a guitar but I haven't played much recently either.'

'We should get together and see how much we can remember. I really enjoyed playing and I miss it.'

'I'd like that. I'll get some new strings on my guitar and see if I can get my fingers moving again.'

'We'll talk about it later. Now come in and meet the crowd. They're a great bunch and we all meet up here every Thursday. You'll find them very friendly.'

The Sportsman Inn was not the most salubrious building I had ever seen. If you were driving around looking for a pub it was probably the sort of place you would choose to avoid on the grounds that it looked a bit seedy and the general décor inside did nothing to change that view. It was in dire need of redecoration with aged paintwork, stained by years of contact with tobacco smoke. I was relieved, though slightly surprised, to see that there wasn't any sawdust on the floor. As we entered, the 'true pub smell' – a combination of beer and cigarettes greeted us.

'Hi Dermot,' called a tall, slim fair-haired young man. 'I'm just buying a round of drinks. What are you having?'

'I'm on orange juice, I'm afraid,' Dermot replied despondently.

'It'll be an early night for you then, Dermot,' replied the young man.

Dermot ignored the comment and introduced me to him.

'Good to see you, Justin, I'm Will. What can I get you to drink?'

'The bitter is superb here, Justin,' Dermot advised. 'John, the landlord, really knows how to look after it.'

'Right, I'll have a pint of bitter then please, Will. Thank you very much.'

Although it was early evening, the pub was buzzing with people, mostly young men, and Dermot seemed to know all of them.

'Will is a GP in a practice not far from here. The well-built chap over there with specs is another GP; his name is Dave. That's Stuart with the curly hair and Harry talking to him; they are both solicitors. The very dark tall one at the bar is Spike; he's a vet and the chap in the suit talking to him is Jack; he's a drug rep.'

At that moment we were joined by two other men each with pint glasses. Dermot introduced me to them. 'This is Patrick who is an orthodontist and Andy who is a financial advisor.'

'There's certainly a wide variety of professionals here tonight,' I commented.

'There's someone representing just about every profession you can think of. If you need advice on anything at all you're likely to be able to find it here,' Patrick remarked. 'Phil over there is a landscape gardener, Steve is in banking, Tom is an estate agent and Dan over there is an electronics engineer. The great thing about it is that everyone is so friendly. This pub seems to be the most unlikely place for such a gathering but the atmosphere is fantastic and the beer's superb.'

'Don't rub it in,' Dermot groaned as he took an unenthusiastic swig of his orange juice. 'You'll find, Justin, that everyone is willing to take their turn to buy drinks but at the same time, no-one will try to force drink on to you if you say you don't want it. They're a great bunch of friends and I really look forward to my Thursday evenings here, even when, like tonight, I can't drink alcohol because I'm driving.'

'We've noticed though, Dermot, that you enjoy yourself a lot more when you can drink alcohol,' said Patrick with a grin.

At that moment, a short, stocky man with a receding hairline wearing a smart shirt and tie entered the bar. 'Good evening, everyone,' he called out.

'Good evening, Brian. Had a good day?' Dermot responded.

'Terrible,' Brian groaned. 'I've seen everything today – ingrowing toenails, housemaid's knee, head lice, explosive diarrhoea, you name it; I've seen it – I need a pint!'

'You'll have gathered that Brian's a GP as well,' Dermot explained. 'He's a great character – just married for the third time and still under forty. His last wife went off with the electrician who came to rewire their house but it didn't take him long to find another.'

'We were saying last week,' said Andy, 'that the one thing all his wives had in common is that they all had enormous backsides. If a woman walks into the pub with a huge backside you'll see his eyes come out like organ stops.'

'It's true,' Patrick added.

I noticed that some of the group were finishing their drinks so I stepped to the bar and asked if I could buy a round but Spike immediately intervened. 'We're not having you buying drinks on your first night here, Justin. This round's on me – what are you having?'

'Thanks, Spike but I really don't mind buying a round.'

'Certainly not, do you want another pint?'

'O.K. thanks very much.'

Spike caught the landlord's eye. 'John, another pint for me and Justin here, and will you see what everyone else wants, and have one yourself? We like to see new faces here, Justin; I hope you'll decide to become a regular.'

At precisely half past eight Dermot drained the last few drops of orange juice from his glass. 'It's time we went now, Justin. I hate to drag you away but my supper will be ready and waiting for me at home.'

'All right, Dermot,' I replied somewhat reluctantly as I was very much enjoying the company and the friendly atmosphere. Everyone had taken the trouble to come over and speak to me and I was made to feel very welcome.

'It's amazing how Dermot has to get back for his supper at eight-thirty when he's driving but when he's not, he's often still here at closing time,' Dan remarked. 'Presumably you'll be included in the driving rota so when it's your turn, be prepared for some late nights.'

'Sorry to drag you away, Justin. What do you think to it; it's a great pub, isn't it? I know it's not exactly smart but the atmosphere in there is fantastic and the beer is the best I have ever tasted.'

'I think it's fabulous, Dermot. Thanks for inviting me.'

'Will you be going again?'

'Most definitely; I'll drive next week if you like.'

'You can if you wish. It would be Chris's turn but I'm sure he'll be delighted to postpone it for a week. If you pick me up first I'll show you where he and Alan live. Now about this music – can I bring my guitar round to your cottage one evening.'

'Sure. What sort of music did you use to play?'

'Sixties pop music – Beatles, Rolling Stones – that sort of thing. How about you?'

'Yes, the same. Buddy Holly, Cliff Richard and the Shadows.'

'Do you play lead?'

'Not really – I played rhythm mostly.'

'Do you think you could play lead, Justin because I'm strictly a rhythm man though I do sing a bit as well but there's no way I could sing and play lead. If we're going to get some sort of band together one of us will have to play lead and it looks as if it is going to have to be you.'

'Do you want to get a band together?'

'I did love playing but we need to find a bass player and a drummer before we can call ourselves a band. In the meantime dust off your guitar and get practising lead and we'll see how we get on.'

CHAPTER FORTY TWO

'I'd feel ridiculous walking around in that, Spencer.' I said indignantly as he handed me a brochure containing colour photographs of handsome young male and pretty female models posing in dental surgery settings for the purpose of advertising the latest in surgical work wear. 'Patients will think we're still wearing our pyjamas.'

'Does it matter what we look like? The important thing is that it will be so much more hygienic than keeping on our outdoor clothes. This is the sort of thing they wear at the hospital and I still can't get over how immaculate everything was there. We have a duty to do everything humanly possible to keep our patients free from infection and I think that this is an important step in that direction.'

'Well I still think it looks ridiculous and in my opinion it will put patients off. I personally think the appeal of this practice is that it doesn't look too clinical. It's sort of homely and welcoming and patients like that. In that brochure, they look as if they've come from outer space.'

'Patients don't really care what we look like as long as we're pleasant to them and don't hurt them. They might be a bit surprised at first but they'll very quickly become used to it. I'm convinced that the time has come for us to move forward. If you look at photographs of modern high-powered dental practices in the dental magazines all the staff are dressed like this.'

'So you're suggesting that we all wear it; nurses as well? I can just imagine Beryl's reaction when you tell her that this is what she'll be wearing at work in future. Wendy might accept it, in fact, she'd probably look good in it but the rest of us would look stupid and I can't wait to see Mr Husslebry's reaction when you appear before him dressed in what to him will look like your pyjamas.'

'I'm sorry, Justin, but you're just going to have to get used to the idea because I know that it's the right way to go. The hospital is obviously at the forefront of infection control and we must follow their example.'

I glanced again at the brochure. 'I can tell you right now, Spencer; I absolutely refuse to walk around the practice in white clogs.'

'They're very sensible because you can slip them on and off without touching them with your hands and I believe they are also very comfortable.'

'Well I wouldn't be seen dead in them. Anyway, do you know how much all this will cost? Each of us will need at least two complete outfits in case one gets messed up, so that adds up to eight, plus clogs for those of you prepared to wear them. I'll bet they aren't cheap.'

'I haven't really looked at the price list yet.' He slid out a white sheet of paper from the back of the brochure and as he examined it, his face slowly changed to match the colour of the paper. 'My God,' he groaned, 'I didn't think they'd cost as much as that.'

'Not so keen on the idea now then, Spencer? I thought you considered infection control to be of paramount importance?'

'Oh well yes, I think it is but this particular range of clothing does seem particularly expensive. Perhaps there's something cheaper on the market; I need to look into it.' He quickly folded the brochure and slipped it into the bottom drawer of his desk.

'By the way, you haven't forgotten it's the Toothplan seminar tomorrow have you, Justin?' My heart sank because I didn't really want to go. Since Spencer mentioned it previously, I had dismissed it from my mind and to be honest, I wasn't very sure what Toothplan was all about. I knew it was some sort of private patient scheme but other than that I was completely ignorant. I suppose I had written it off as being another of Spencer's big ideas which, like most of his others, would turn out to be an utter disaster. He had given me some literature which I had merely scanned without gleaning any real understanding but my initial reaction was that the whole thing appeared to be based on American principles which didn't appeal to me. I gathered that the seminar would involve a good deal of role play and audience participation which was another reason why I was dreading it. I wouldn't have minded so much if it had been simply a day of lectures that I could just sit and listen to but I knew that this seminar wasn't going to be like that and I wasn't looking forward to it one little bit.

'It's being held at the Crown Hotel so the lunch should be good,' said Spencer, sensing my lack of enthusiasm.

'What time does it start?'

'Ten o'clock, which will give you ample time to get there, Justin, without you having to set off too early.'

'Won't we be going there together? There's no point in taking two cars.'

Spencer started to look shifty. 'Ah, well,' he stammered. 'I'm afraid I shan't be able to go after all – I'm very disappointed about it.'

'I'll bet you are, Spencer! Why can't you go?'

'Pressure of work.'

'Don't give me that! You said that you'd get Beryl to cross off the day in your appointment book, so what happened?'

'I had so many patients asking for appointments, I had to cancel the seminar to fit them in.'

'Frankly, I find that very hard to believe! You never had any intention of going in the first place. Show me your appointment book – let's see how busy you are.'

'There's no need to get upset, Justin but I really do think it would be irresponsible for us to close the practice down completely for the day. One of us needs to be here to deal with any emergencies and as I thought you were keen to go to the seminar I phoned up and cancelled my reservation so that I could stay here and hold the fort.'

'That's very magnanimous of you! Whatever gave you the idea I was keen? I haven't even mentioned it. If you want the truth, I haven't the slightest inclination to go.'

Before Spencer could say another word, I snatched his appointment book off his desk. 'You've got three patients all day! So where are all these patients asking for appointments?'

'As I said, Justin, someone needs to be here to hold the fort.'

'In that case, I'll stay here and you can go to the seminar in my place.'

'I would but Mr Phillips is coming in tomorrow so that I can finish his treatment before he goes on holiday at the weekend; I can't let him down now the appointment has been made. But I do think it's important for us to find out more about Toothplan because I think a private patient scheme will be good for the practice so one of us should go and unfortunately, it can't be me now, so it will have to be you.'

'Yes it is unfortunate – it's unfortunate for me.'

'I'm sure you'll enjoy it when you get there and as I said, at least you'll get a good lunch.'

'Food isn't as important to me as it obviously is to you, Spencer,' I quipped somewhat truculently. He ignored my remark and started rooting around on his desk.

'There's no more to be said, Justin. One of us has to be there for the good of the practice and, unfortunately, it can't be me because I'm committed here so that's the end of the matter. Changing the subject, I've had a letter from the hospital about Mr Jolly and it's not good news, I'm afraid – he's got leukaemia.'

'That's terrible; can they do anything for him?'

'Oh yes, they're beginning treatment right away and there is a good chance that he'll be all right. Luckily it was caught early.'

'That's thanks to you, Spencer.'

'I was only doing my job. It just proves that we have an important part to play in monitoring our patients for this sort of problem; we need to be constantly on the lookout.'

'I hope he'll be all right; he seems such a nice chap.'

'I hope so too, Justin. Now I really must get on.'

'I know; pressure of work prevents you from wasting any more time chatting to me!'

I too needed to get back to my surgery because I was aware that Mrs Newman would be coming in very shortly for me to see how she was getting on with her new crowns. I was more than a little apprehensive as I felt sure that she would realise by now that she had made a mistake and that her crowns were far too big. I was dreading the prospect of having to remove them in order to get them remade. I tried to console myself with the thought that perhaps she would have been back sooner had she been really unhappy and I began to feel a lot better when Wendy came in waving a cheque in front of my nose. 'Yes, she's paid in full and I think you need to prepare yourself for a surprise,' was all she would say.

I hardly recognised Mrs Newman. The dowdy clothes had been replaced with a vibrant and fashionable new outfit, she had changed the style and colour of her hair and must have spent hours applying her make-up. The transformation was unbelievable; she looked positively glamorous but what struck me more than anything was that she seemed to have adapted perfectly to her new crowns. They were very much on display because she was smiling in a way that she had never done before but remarkably, they didn't look at all oversized.

'I love your new surgery, Mr Derwent,' were her opening words.

'Thank you, Mrs Newman, but never mind my surgery, what about the new you!'

'I can't thank you enough, Mr Derwent you have changed my life in a way that I never thought possible. I feel a completely different woman.'

'You look like a different woman if you don't mind my saying so.'

'I just wish I'd had my teeth done years ago, but we can't put the clock back so I shall just have to make up for lost time as quickly as I can.'

'I'm so delighted that it has worked out so well, Mrs Newman. I must admit I had grave reservations about changing your smile in the way that we have. There's no doubt you were right and I was wrong about it.'

'I knew what I wanted and I'm so grateful to you for giving it to me. I'll come and see you in about six months to get everything checked if that's all right with you.'

She had only just gone through the door when Beryl came out of the office. 'Justin, I've got Dr Fitzpatrick on the phone for you.'

'Good morning, Dermot.'

He sounded very excited. 'Justin, I think I've found us a bass player. He's a GP and has played bass for many years – he's apparently very good and has on occasions played with some famous bands.'

'Sounds as though he might be a bit too good for us, Dermot; certainly too good for me. Does he know that we haven't actually played together yet and that neither of us has played seriously for many years?'

'I've just been speaking to him and I merely said that you and I are thinking of getting together to form a band. I didn't go into detail at this stage about the fact that we haven't played much for some time. Anyway he said he'd be very happy to come and play with us and see how we get on. I've stalled him for the present so what we need to do is to sort out a few numbers and work like mad on them together until we can play them well, then we'll get him round. We won't tell him we've practised; we'll let him think that it's ages since we picked up a guitar and we're just playing from memory so he won't be expecting much from us, then if we sound quite good, hopefully he'll be impressed and might be prepared to stick with us.'

'How well do you know him?'

'I've only met him a couple of times at medical functions but I've heard quite a lot about him though I didn't know he plays bass until my receptionist told me. As soon as I heard that I phoned him. He's a great big chap – must be six feet four at least and well-built. Everyone calls him 'Big Tone'. His name is Tony and he's called 'big Tone' obviously because of his size but apparently, according to my receptionist, he acquired the name partly because his bass playing can be a bit loud. He's definitely not the sort of chap to stand for any nonsense though I mean that in a complimentary way. His patients think the world of him because he's very caring and he moves heaven and earth to make sure they get the best possible care if he refers them on. Apparently the consultants at the hospital are scared to death of him because he expects results quickly and he keeps on at them until they deliver. What do you think? It's worth giving him a try, isn't it?

'He sounds pretty formidable; we'd better make sure we're good before we invite him round to join us.'

'Oh absolutely, Justin. Now I'll let you get on, meanwhile I've got to see if I can find us a drummer.'

CHAPTER FORTY THREE

I was feeling quite gloomy as the last patient left my surgery. The elation of achieving a successful outcome with Mrs Newman was not enough to overcome my dismay at the prospect of going to the Toothplan seminar next day and I was also missing Harriet. She sometimes phoned me in the evening but I hadn't heard from her for a few days and I was beginning to feel a bit concerned. I still wasn't sure about her feelings for me and I was aware that at university she would be surrounded by many hot-blooded young male students and after all, she was very attractive. I felt sure she would receive a lot of attention which troubled me greatly. I tried to dismiss it from my thoughts but there were times when I found it difficult. It was a wonderful surprise, therefore, when the patients' bell rang and it was her standing on the doorstep.

'Harriet, how lovely to see you.' I hugged her and we kissed.

'I'm sorry I didn't phone,' she said, 'but I wanted to surprise you. I thought you would still be here. Are you working?'

'No my last patient has just left. It's wonderful to see you; come into the kitchen and I'll make you a cup of tea.'

'I'm pleased to be back here,' she sighed, 'I really don't like Southampton. How are you getting on?'

'All right, but I'm not looking forward to tomorrow; Spencer's conned me into going to a seminar to do with a private patient scheme. He was supposed to be going with me but he's skived off at the last minute so I shall be going on my own.'

'Well it will make a change from being stuck in the surgery; you might actually enjoy it.'

'I doubt it – it's all sounds a bit too interactive for my liking. There's going to be a lot of role play and audience participation, which I find a bit pointless.'

'It could be fun.'

'It's not my idea of fun. I wouldn't mind if it consisted of lectures by someone who knows what they're talking about but I've absolutely no desire to make a fool of myself or see other people make fools of themselves by indulging in role play. I don't learn anything from it and I see it as a complete waste of time. I don't know who devised this method of conducting seminars but they are very misguided if they think it's effective.'

'It was psychologists, actually, Justin.'

I couldn't help laughing. 'You lot?'

'I'm not sure I qualify as belonging to that elite group just yet but yes it was psychologists who decided that people learn much more effectively if they are involved. After all, you must admit that it's very easy to switch off in a lecture and learn absolutely nothing from it.'

'Well, true, and I can understand that if you're dealing with children it's important to keep them interested and attentive but surely adults can make their own minds up whether they want to learn or not and they don't expect to be treated like five-year-olds.'

'Research has shown that by adopting these techniques there's a better chance of imparting knowledge whether it's with children or adults and don't forget it's expensive to run a course so this is more cost effective. After all, you don't want it to be a complete waste of money and have people coming away without learning anything.'

'Oh of course; everything's about money these days.'

'I'm afraid it is. Anyway you'll have to get used to being taught in this way because more and more organisations are adopting this approach.'

'In that case I shall attend as few courses as possible. The good, old-fashioned lecture worked for me at university and I can't see any need to change.'

Our conversation was interrupted when the patients' bell rang again. I left Harriet in the kitchen and went to answer it. You can imagine my surprise and consternation to see Sarah standing there.

'I'm glad I caught you before you went home, Justin but my mother wanted me to give you this letter.'

I took it from her and briefly glanced at it before placing it on the table in the entrance hall. I could see it was to thank me for helping with her serving hatch 'Thank you, Sarah.' I said looking behind me to see if Harriet had remained in the kitchen, 'but she thanked me at the time; she didn't need to write to me.'

'She wanted to; she was so grateful for your help. Aren't you going to invite me in and show me your new surgery?'

'Oh yes, I'm sorry, do come in.' I stepped aside to let her enter and at that moment Harriet emerged from the kitchen. 'This is Harriet; Harriet meet Sarah.'

The two girls shook hands and seemed amicably disposed towards each other but I was beginning to perspire and decided it might be expedient to separate them. 'Come and look at my surgery, Sarah; it seems to be working well and I'm so pleased to have the new equipment.' I was relieved when Harriet did not follow us but remained in the entrance hall drinking her tea.

After what seemed like an eternity but was probably only about ten minutes, Sarah decided that she had stayed long enough. She obviously wasn't expecting to find me with another girl and possibly felt almost as uncomfortable as I did. 'Thank you for showing me your surgery, Justin; it looks fabulous. Now I really must be getting back.'

I showed her out and breathed a sigh of relief as I returned to the kitchen where Harriet was sitting at the table. 'I'm sorry about that Harriet; I had no idea she was going to turn up.'

'What did she want?' Harriet demanded sharply.

'She came to deliver a letter from her mother. It was to thank me for something I did for her some time ago. Apparently she'd been meaning to write to me for some time but has only just got around to it.'

'Is that so?' said Harriet doubtfully. I could feel my temperature beginning to rise again as the feeling of relief I had experienced when Sarah left, began to dissolve away. Harriet looked at me with her piercing blue eyes which were so beautiful but at that moment so intimidating. I felt an overwhelming urge to look away but I knew that I was under psychological scrutiny and looking away would not be at all wise.

'I know that you've seen Sarah recently so don't deny it, Justin.'

I realised there was no point in going on trying to deceive her any further so I attempted to adopt a damage limitation approach. I also knew that it would be pointless to start pouring out excuses because she would see straight through them so I decided to say as little as possible and to parry each blow as it came. I tried desperately to think logically and came to the conclusion that she couldn't possibly know for sure that I'd seen Sarah; she was just calling my bluff.

'What makes you say that?' I replied, feeling confident that she would not be able to provide concrete evidence that proved my guilt. Her reply shattered me.

'Whilst you were showing Sarah your surgery, I read her mother's letter so I know you've been to her house.'

'You read her letter? That's a despicable thing to do, Harriet. I'm really shocked to know you would do that. It was a private letter and you had absolutely no right to read it.'

'It's lucky for me that I did because you weren't going to tell me you'd seen her, were you? You were going to deceive me, Justin.'

'I only went to their house to help create a serving hatch. Sarah's mother asked me and I felt sorry for her and didn't feel I could say no but that's all there was to it; I swear to you.'

'Well if it was all so innocent, why didn't you tell me?'

'Because I didn't want you to think there was still something between Sarah and me and I wasn't sure you'd understand. I thought it best to keep quiet about it so as not to upset you.'

'Well you've upset me now.'

'You've upset me too, Harriet. I can't believe that you would have the nerve to read my private correspondence; it's a disgraceful thing to do and I'm utterly shocked that you could do it. It's absolutely unforgiveable.'

'It would be if I really had read the letter but actually, I didn't; I wouldn't do that, Justin, I was just bluffing. I said I'd read it in the belief that if you thought I had, you wouldn't try to hide the truth from me anymore.'

'But you said that you knew I'd seen Sarah recently. How could you have known that if you didn't read the letter?'

'I didn't for sure, but what made me suspicious was that she never mentioned your new car. It's parked right outside so she couldn't have missed seeing it. The fact that she didn't say anything about it suggested to me that she'd already seen it before.'

'So why did you say that you'd read the letter? Why didn't you just say that you knew Sarah and I must have met because she didn't mention my car?'

'It would have been too easy for you to say that you'd just bumped into each other by chance somewhere and that's how she knew about your car. I've no idea what's in the letter but I played a hunch by saying that I'd read it and that it told me that you had been to see her. It worked, didn't it, because it made you spill the beans and come clean?'

'How devious can you get?' I replied indignantly.

'Devious? I like that, Justin! You were the one who was being devious by not telling me that you'd been to meet Sarah. I'm very disappointed in you because I thought you were honest and straight.'

She stood up and walked out leaving me feeling very upset and annoyed. I'm not sure whether I was annoyed with her for trapping me like that or whether I was annoyed with myself for being stupid enough to try and deceive her. If I'd been open with her from the start then maybe none of this would have happened. All I knew was that I felt annoyed and even gloomier than previously now that Harriet had walked out on me.

CHAPTER FORTY FOUR

The seminar was every bit as bad as I had feared. The fact that I was so distraught about Harriet made it a hundred times worse and I found it very difficult to concentrate. She had said that the interactive method of teaching is a more effective way of imparting knowledge. All I can say is that on this occasion it failed miserably as I came away with only the faintest idea of what it had all been about. When I arrived at the surgery next morning, Spencer pounced on me and couldn't wait to ask me about it.

'If you're so interested, Spencer, why didn't you go yourself; then you'd know?' I said grumpily. 'It was all so puerile; I couldn't be bothered to listen most of the time. I learnt absolutely nothing about how Toothplan works. In fact, it seems that the course wasn't about that; its purpose was to instruct us on how to sell it to our patients.'

'I could have told you that,' Spencer replied haughtily, 'and if you'd taken the time to read the leaflet you'd have known too. That's one of the reasons, apart from pressure of work, of course, why I didn't go because I didn't think I would get a lot out of it. I'm perfectly capable of selling something to my patients without having to go on courses to learn how to do it, whereas, you, with all due respect, might not find it quite so easy. That's why I thought the course would be beneficial for you. There's a meeting early next week when the managing director of Toothplan will be telling us exactly how the scheme works. That will be a useful meeting and we'll both definitely be going.'

'I shall really look forward to it,' I said sarcastically.

'What's the matter with you today, Justin; you seem very depressed about something.'

'Oh nothing, Spencer.'

'Surely the course wasn't that upsetting was it? Tell me about it.'

'It was absolutely stupid from start to finish. We kicked off by pairing up with the person next to us and we each had two minutes to tell the other one as much as possible about ourselves and our background. Then we had to stand up in turn and tell the group what we knew about our partner. It was a complete disaster because people were getting things wrong most of the time so the person being talked about had to keep butting in to put the record straight. In any case, nobody listened because everyone was too preoccupied with trying to remember what they were going to say when it was their turn to speak and when you'd done your bit you were so relieved to get it over with you just switched off completely so the whole thing was a total waste of time. God knows why we couldn't have just introduced ourselves.'

The next hour was spent writing our own mission statement which was also a completely pointless exercise as far as I could see. It was just words. Do the idiots who organise these courses honestly think that stringing a few words together to say how we intend to dedicate ourselves towards providing the highest standard of treatment for our patients is actually going to influence the way we think and behave or that any of our patients believe a word of it? They'll judge you as a dentist by the treatment they receive from you not by something you've written. And as a dentist; either you want to do the best for your patients or you don't and writing a fatuous mission statement is not going to change things.'

'So what was your mission statement?' queried Spencer with a mischievous chuckle.

'To get away from this ludicrous seminar as quickly as possible.'

'I'll bet they were impressed by that! So what came next?'

'Some nerd stood up and started telling us how we should improve our practice image – flowers in the waiting room, attractive pictures on the walls, make sure your receptionist smiles a lot – that sort of thing; all highly innovative, earthshattering ideas that nobody has ever even dreamed about before.'

Spencer just smiled and waited for me to continue to get it all off my chest.

'The crowning glory was in the afternoon when we were expected to engage in role play. One of us pretended to be the patient and someone else had to take on the role of the dentist going through the process of selling Toothplan to them. I was teamed up with some pretentious oaf who tried to be as difficult as he could be and did his best to make me look an idiot by asking all sorts of questions which I couldn't answer. I was in a bad mood before I went to the seminar but I can tell you; it just about finished me.'

'Justin, Justin; calm yourself down. What is the matter with you? Is there something troubling you? You're normally so placid; it's not like you to get yourself all worked up like this.'

I didn't really want to tell him that I was feeling down because of Harriet. He already thought that my love life was a bit of a joke and I wasn't going to give him reason to expand his opinion. I could also tell from the way he was smirking that he considered my ranting and raving about the seminar to be highly amusing. 'It's nothing, Spencer, now I must get on.'

Beryl popped her head round the door. 'Spencer, Mr Dickson's in the waiting room – he wants to see you.'

'Isn't that the chap whose tooth you extracted at the hospital?' I enquired.

'Yes it is. I wonder what he wants.'

Once I started work I began to feel a bit calmer though I found it difficult to get Harriet out of my mind. I felt very foolish for not telling her that I had been to help Sarah's mother but it was too late now; the damage was done. I was wondering what course of action I should take to try to remedy the situation because I was too fond of her to let her slip away from me that easily when Beryl came in to tell me that Dermot was on the phone wanting to speak to me.

'Hi Justin, I'm just phoning to say that I might possibly have found us a drummer though I'm not really sure whether he would be any good. He's a doctor at the hospital and used to play drums a little bit many years ago though he says he never really learnt to play well. I'm a bit concerned because he seems to flit around a lot and never seems to stay in one place for very long, which could be a problem. Also he doesn't actually own any drums.'

'Doesn't sound too promising, Dermot.'

'Well no but I was wondering if it would be a good idea for us to buy a drum kit between us. It needn't be anything fancy, just a second hand kit which we could probably pick up fairly cheaply and if we find someone who might be interested in playing with us, like this chap, we could lend them the drums to see how they get on. If it doesn't work out we take them back. I also wondered if this chap isn't any good whether your girlfriend, Harriet, might be interested in learning. It would be good to have a female drummer.'

'I'm not sure she's my girlfriend any more – we had a bit of a disagreement.'

'Oh that's a shame; she seemed nice but you need to choose carefully – if you make a mistake with your woman it can have serious consequences. Anyway, it was just a thought. Oh, by the way, Big Tone is longing to come and play with us; he phoned up again to see when we can get together. I'm still putting him off but I can't keep on doing it; we need to get practising.'

'I'm tied up for a few days, Dermot, but I'll ring you early next week.'

'O.K. Justin, take care.'

Dermot certainly seemed to be taking the idea of forming a band very seriously and I was quite enthusiastic too but at the moment, Harriet was dominating my thoughts and I found it difficult to focus my attention on anything else. I returned to my surgery where I had been in the process of scaling Mrs Drummond's horse-like teeth. She didn't seem to mind that I had left her to answer the phone and was happily chatting to Wendy. I felt, however, that it might be stretching her tolerance to the limit when Beryl came in to tell me that there was another phone call for me.

'Who is it this time?'

'It's someone called Michael from Toothplan.'

'Hello.'

'Dr Derwent?'

Doctor, I thought. Either my status has suddenly risen unexpectedly or someone's trying to butter me up. 'Yes, speaking.'

'Hello, Dr Derwent, my name's Michael and I'm your Toothplan Local Liaison Manager. I understand you attended our seminar yesterday, did you find it beneficial?'

'To be perfectly honest, I'm not sure that I did.'

'Really? You do surprise me because the feedback from most dentists is that they think it is very instructive and informative, and enjoyable too. What was it that wasn't to your liking?'

'I felt I was being treated like a child in kindergarten; I'd have preferred to have listened to lectures by accomplished speakers instead of having to engage in the various activities, such as role play.'

'But it's been proved that this is a far more effective way of teaching, however, we are of course, always ready to listen to different

285

views. I'm very sorry that you didn't enjoy the day because a lot of thought and planning went into organising it. I'm sure you probably benefitted from it more than you realise and the skills you acquired will be very useful if, and I sincerely hope you will, sign up to Toothplan. I mustn't detain you because we at Toothplan are aware that you dentists are extremely busy people and I don't want to keep you from your patients a moment longer than is necessary but the main reason I'm phoning is to ask if you were given a copy of the Toothplan song yesterday.'

'The what?'

'The Toothplan song. It's the song we always sing together at the start of our main meetings – we'll certainly be singing it at the start of the meeting on Tuesday evening, which I understand you will be attending with Mr Padginton.'

'No I wasn't given a copy of it.'

'But you will be attending the meeting?'

'Yes,' I sighed.

'Good, in that case it's important that you get a copy of the song before the meeting so that you can familiarise yourself with it and join in the singing. We believe that singing a song together helps to put everyone into the right frame of mind and prepares them to unite together in a common cause which is, of course, Toothplan. You'll find the words of the song very stimulating. I'll post a copy to you if I get time but if not, I'll arrange for you to be given a copy as soon as you arrive at the meeting. I very much look forward to seeing you on Tuesday. Bye for now and have a good day.'

'Arghh,' I groaned, 'how I hate that expression,' but after yesterday, it's exactly what I would expect someone from Toothplan to say.

I went back to my surgery and finished Mrs Drummond's scaling. After she'd left I couldn't wait to find Spencer. 'Well that just about takes the biscuit. Did you know that there's a Toothplan song which they sing at the start of all their meetings?'

'Er, yes I think I did, Justin,' Spencer replied casually.

'Well don't you think it's a stupid idea?'

'I haven't really thought about it but if that's what they want to do I can't see anything wrong with it.'

I exploded. 'You can't see anything wrong with it? Spencer, the whole thing is an absolute joke! The more I learn about Toothplan and their way of doing things, the more it gets right up my nose. It strikes me as being very American in its concept, it's cheap, tacky, cheesy, tasteless, and I hate it!'

'Don't get yourself so steamed up, Justin. It's true that they don't operate quite in the way that we've been used to but things move on. Toothplan is a relatively new idea and I'm beginning to think that their approach is modern and original and perhaps it's time we loosened up and accepted the change. Let's just go along with it and see how it works out; there's no point in fighting it.'

'I can't believe you've just said that, Spencer; what's happening to you? You were always the last person to accept change but now you seem to have adopted an entirely different mind-set.'

'I don't think you can say that just because I'm prepared to reserve judgement on Toothplan.'

'What about all this infection control business, you've been on about ever since you went to the hospital to extract Mr Dickson's tooth?'

'Ah well, I might have had a bit of a rethink on that one.'

'That's because you saw how expensive it would be to kit us all out in surgical attire.'

'It isn't actually, Justin. Mr Dickson came to see me this morning in agony – the fact is – he's got an infected socket!'

'I don't believe it; after all that infection control at the hospital? It just goes to show doesn't it?'

'It certainly does.'

CHAPTER FORTY FIVE

'I really don't understand, Mr Newman,' I stammered, wincing as the pain in my ribs intensified with each additional jab from a rock-hard finger which was now feeling more like a battering ram. 'I can assure you that my relationship with your wife has been entirely professional.'

'Really? Well this professional relationship as you call it has caused me nothing but trouble.'

'I don't see how. I simply carried out some treatment for her and when I saw her very recently she seemed happy with it. What exactly is the problem?'

'She might be happy but I'm bloody well not. We were getting along just fine until you came on the scene. She was no great beauty but that didn't bother me; I'm no oil painting either, but after you'd finished with her, she seemed to think that suddenly she'd become a bloody glamour puss.'

'Isn't it good that she's concerned about her appearance? Lots of women want to look good for their husbands; aren't you pleased that she's made the effort for you?'

'It's not for me! She used to do my washing, clean the house and have my dinner ready when I got home from work and I was happy with that but now she's never in. I never know when I'm going to see her or when I'm going to get my next meal. She stays out half the night, spends a fortune on clothes make-up and hair-dos, which she never did before, not to mention the extortionate amount of money you charged for doing her teeth. I'm bloody well paying for all this because she doesn't work. You started all this by persuading her to have her teeth done.'

'I can assure you that I didn't persuade her; it was entirely her decision to have the work done on her teeth. In fact, to begin with, I didn't think it was a very good idea and I tried to talk her out of it.'

'Oh, really?' scoffed Mr Newman. 'I find that very hard to believe. I bet you couldn't wait to get your sweaty little hands on her, or rather my money.'

'It wasn't like that. It was completely her idea; she knew exactly what she wanted and there was nothing I could do or say to change her views. I'm sure if I hadn't done it for her she would have gone to another dentist. I still think that deep down she did it because it would please you.'

'Well if it was for me, how do you explain the fact that she's gone and found herself a bloody toy boy? She's old enough to be his mother but according to her, they're madly in love. They can't keep their hands off each other and it makes me sick to see it. It's bloody disgusting – she's behaving like a stupid, love-sick teenager.'

'It's probably only a temporary blip. She suddenly feels good about herself and her appearance and at the moment she's letting off steam. She's probably dreamed about looking attractive for many years and now that she's achieved it she doesn't quite know how to handle it.'

I was struggling to put together a plausible psychological assessment which would hopefully help to calm Mr Newman down and I felt sure that Harriet would have done a much better job of it. At the moment I just wanted to say something that would persuade him to stop banging my head against the door.

'I'm sure,' I continued, 'it won't last long. She'll come to her senses if you just give her a bit of time and space. She'll soon get tired of this young man and come back to you.'

'I doubt it. She's told me she wants a divorce so she must be serious.'

'She's said that but I doubt if she really means it.'

'You haven't seen how she's carrying on – she means it all right. I'm not so bothered about her leaving me; I can cope with that but what I can't accept is that she's determined to claim half of everything I've worked for over the past twelve years. She's no money of her own and hasn't worked since we got married so it seems bloody unfair that she can now claim half of everything. It's tantamount to theft especially as it's going to line the pockets of some snotty-nosed little brat who's got his grubby little claws into her. The novelty will soon wear off when he realises he's landed himself with a middle-aged woman who's nowhere near as exciting as he thought she was and he'll drop her like a hot potato but by then he'll have got hold of my money.'

'I'm sorry for you, Mr Newman. It seems grossly unfair but that's the way the law works and divorces are always messy affairs. I don't see how I can be held responsible for her wanting a divorce though.'

I felt his grip on my throat tighten and I rather gathered that this was probably not a sensible thing to say. Again I wondered how Harriet would have handled the situation though I suspected that Mr Newman would not have been quite so physical if I had been a woman.

'Please take your hand off my throat and stop digging me in the ribs, Mr Newman, and let's talk about this in a civilised way. I'm truly sorry about the way things have worked out but I'm not sure there's anything I can do about it. What do you want from me and why did you come to see me today?'

'I came to knock the hell out of you for creating this mess.'

'That might make you feel better in the short term but it won't alter the situation between you and your wife.'

'I suppose not but I'm just so angry.'

'I can understand that.' Mercifully, he let go of me and suddenly his enormous stature appeared to diminish 'but I really don't see what I can do to help.'

'There is one thing you could do to make amends.'

'I will if I can but I don't honestly see how. What do you have in mind?'

'Well look at my teeth; they look terrible. They're crooked and stained and I wondered if you could crown them like you did my wife's.'

'Yes, I'm sure that could be done. If you'd like to arrange an appointment I'll take some X-rays and carry out a full assessment.'

'Really, that's good. If it has the same effect on me as it did on my wife I might even find myself a young bit of stuff to keep me company during the cold winter nights. All right, I'll make an appointment. There is one other condition though – you have to do it free of charge.'

I gulped at the financial implications as I would have to pay a technician to make the crowns and it would be an expensive exercise for me but at that moment I was so relieved to escape unscathed from a potential physical attack that I considered it unwise to argue with him. I didn't agree or disagree to his request.

'If you see Wendy, she'll make an appointment for you.'

Spencer never seemed to be very far away at times like this and had heard most of the conversation though I noticed that he had made no attempt to step in and save me from being beaten up. He was grinning broadly as he approached.

'Sounds like a case of new teeth in her head – new man in her bed!' he quipped. 'It's an amazing coincidence that her name is "Newman".'

CHAPTER FORTY SIX

Spencer had kindly offered to drive us to the Toothplan meeting. The whole practice team was invited so poor Beryl and Wendy received orders from Spencer that they had to attend as well. The arrangement was that he would collect them before picking me up at around six o'clock. I was pacing around waiting for him, wondering how to pass the time then suddenly on impulse I decided to telephone Harriet.

I had been thinking about her a great deal and going over in my mind the events which took place the last time we were together. I had reached the conclusion that I didn't really have any cause to be annoyed with her because she hadn't actually done anything wrong. It's true that I got angry when I thought she had read the letter from Sarah's mother but I'm sure now that she didn't really read it – she just said she had and I could see why she said it. She caught me very neatly in a well thought out trap and, looking back on it, it was very clever of her and I had to admire her lively thinking, even if it was rather cunning. I, on the other hand, had not been open with her. I should have told her that I had seen Sarah and explained the circumstances. It was stupid of me to try to deceive her and if, as I was hoping, Harriet had contemplated a serious relationship with me it would not have improved my chances when she found out I had been to see an ex-girlfriend behind her back. I couldn't let her slip away from me because my feelings for her were deeper and stronger than anything I had ever experienced before and I had come to realise that I loved her.

My heart was pounding as I waited anxiously for my phone call to be answered. I knew immediately that the voice at the other end belonged to Harriet's mother.

'Hello, Mrs Brooks, it's Justin Derwent here. Is Harriet there by any chance?'

'I'm afraid she's not, Justin; she's gone out with a boy from university who lives not far from here. He's asked her out several times before and she's always said no but this time she accepted his invitation to go out for a drink.'

Her words hit me like a thunderbolt and I felt insanely jealous. For a moment I was unable to speak.

'Are you still there, Justin?' Mrs Brooks asked.

'Err, yes I'm still here. Will you tell her I phoned?'

'Yes though I don't know what time she'll be back. Do you want me to get her to phone you?'

'Err, no it doesn't matter. Good bye.'

'Good bye, Justin.'

I felt utterly deflated and devastated. My feeling of jealousy was soon overwhelmed by intense pangs of anger with myself for allowing the situation to occur in the first place. Harriet must have had feelings for me otherwise why would she have come to see me as soon as she got back from university, so finding out I had not been open with her must have upset her. The burning question in my mind now was whether she had gone out with someone else because she had decided that she and I had no future together or whether she was doing it simply to make me jealous. Perhaps it was another example of psychology in action.

Spencer's arrival prevented me from indulging in further analysis and reluctantly I jumped into the car beside him with Beryl and Wendy in the back seat. Attending a Toothplan meeting was just about the last thing I wanted to do at that moment but strangely, the other three seemed unnaturally enthusiastic about it.

'Should be very interesting,' Spencer effused.

'I'm glad you think so, Spencer. I can't think of anything worse at this moment.'

'I'm sure it's the way forward for our practice.' He continued. 'I know some of our patients are already private as opposed to national health but this could be the way to convert a good many more.'

'It certainly sounds a good scheme,' Beryl added. 'What do you think about it, Justin?'

'The scheme itself might be all right though I'm reserving judgement until after tonight's meeting,' I replied gloomily. 'I certainly didn't enjoy the seminar I went to; I thought it was a complete waste of time and energy.'

'What's the matter with you, Justin?' Spencer responded. 'You've been moody and miserable for the past few days. Have you got woman trouble again?'

'Not exactly,' I lied.

'Not exactly? Then I think we can safely assume that you have. You don't seem to do very well with women, Justin, I don't know why it is but you always seem to finish up in trouble.'

'Can we change the subject, Spencer; I don't want to talk about it.'

'All right we'll talk about tonight's meeting. Have you got your copy of the Toothplan song?'

'Oh don't start that again. No I haven't got a copy of it and I think the idea of singing an inane song before every meeting is just about the last straw as far as I'm concerned.'

'There you go again, getting yourself all steamed up. It's only a song, Justin.'

Beryl and Wendy chimed in. 'Yes it will be fun to sing a song to get us all into a good frame of mind; we're looking forward to it.'

'Well, I'm not and I certainly shan't be singing. If *you* want to, that's up to you but leave me out of it and if there's any repeat of the silly behaviour I had to endure at the seminar I shall leave.'

'Well you won't get far,' Spencer chuckled, 'I'm driving. You'll have to wait until the end of the meeting before you can go home so you might as well sit it out. In any case, we're going to learn how the scheme works so it's important for you to listen and learn. And for goodness sake cheer up; it might do you good to join in a good rousing song.'

We arrived with time to spare before the meeting was due to start. 'Why don't you, Wendy and Beryl go and get some coffee for us and I'll join you in a minute. I'm just going to pop into the lecture room to make sure our seats have been reserved.'

The way I was feeling indicated that something considerably stronger than coffee would have been more welcome but unfortunately they didn't serve alcohol. Spencer soon came to sit with us. 'We have some good seats right at the front,' he announced, much to my dismay as I would have much preferred to sit inconspicuously at the back. I secretly strengthened my resolve to get up and leave at the first hint of audience participation.

We drank our coffee and Spencer led us into the lecture room. 'There are our seats over there,' he pointed. 'There appears to be an envelope addressed to you on that seat, Justin.'

'Oh my God,' I thought, 'it's the bloody Toothplan song. Michael said he would make sure I had a copy before the meeting – I thought he'd forgotten about it.'

I looked at the envelope on which was neatly typed:

URGENT   *For the attention of Dr J. Derwent*

I tore it open to find enclosed, a letter on official Toothplan headed notepaper which read:

Dear Dr Derwent

I am sorry that you have not yet received a copy of the Toothplan song which is, of course sung at the start of all Toothplan meetings. I haven't had the chance to get this in the post to you and have, therefore, copied the words out. I hope you enjoy the meeting tonight.

Yours sincerely

Michael from Toothplan

THE TOOTHPLAN SONG

(To the tune of Oh Dear What Can the Matter Be?)

If your practice is failing
There's no point in moaning and wailing
Listen to what our team is unveiling
And sign up to Toothplan today

Your bank manager won't feel the need for curtailing
The time that you spend on your golfing and sailing
You'll even enjoy doing fillings and scalings
So sign up to Toothplan today

Difficult patients like old Mr Husslebry
Those who you dread 'cause you know what a fuss there'll be
No longer make you rush to the lavatory
Sign up to Toothplan today

With Wendy and Beryl and Spencer beside you
And Michael from Toothplan whose job is to guide you
And no NHS regulations to chide you
Sign up to Toothplan today

Come forward you dentists and let us unite
With Toothplan behind you the future looks bright
The riches you've dreamed of will soon be in sight
So sign up to Toothplan today.

I looked across at Spencer who was trying to hide his face behind a piece of paper which was too small to be effective. I could see that he was splitting his sides with laughter. Beryl and Wendy were sharing the mirth. 'The three of you are in it together,' I exclaimed. 'And you, Spencer or should I say *Michael from Toothplan,* are an absolute swine for winding me up like that.'

'I said I would get even with you for the trick you played on me in connection with my X-ray machine. I reckon it's fifteen all now.'

CHAPTER FORTY SEVEN

The meeting was nowhere near as bad as I had feared, in fact, it turned out to be quite interesting taking the form of a talk by the managing director of Toothplan in which he explained how the scheme worked. Afterwards he invited questions from the audience and Spencer and I came away thinking that it would be good for our practice and well worth considering. Mercifully, there was no singing before the meeting.

Spencer did not gloat about the fact that he had successfully played a clever trick on me by winding me up about the Toothplan song and once he had established that he had evened the score with respect to the prank I played on him over his X-ray machine, he was happy to let the matter rest. I suspect he spared my feelings because he was aware that my love life was in disarray and although I didn't go into details about my disagreement with Harriet, he knew that I was fond of her and could understand why I was downhearted.

I had hoped that she might telephone me in response to my call to her mother but several days went by and I still hadn't heard from her though perhaps she was waiting for me to make another attempt to get in touch. By Saturday morning I was beside myself with disappointment that she hadn't made contact; with grief that our relationship might be over; with jealously at the thought she had been out with someone else; with anger at my own stupidity for not being open with her; and uncertainty as to how best to try and resolve matters. My mind was in turmoil but I was certain of one thing; I couldn't just let her slip out of my life without making some effort to get her back.

Drastic action was called for and after much soul searching I decided upon a course of action which was extremely exciting though slightly scary. A favourable outcome would see me ecstatic but if it didn't work out I would be left in the depths of despair; I just hoped I had the nerve to see it through.

I picked up the phone and dialled Harriet's number. To my great relief, it was she and not her mother who answered.

'Hello Justin, what a pleasant surprise, how are you?'

'Not too bad thanks, Harriet. How are you?'

'Yes I'm all right but it hasn't been a very good week. I had some essays to write which took up a lot of time. I intended writing them at home but I soon realised I would need the university library for research so I had to go back to Southampton. I'm sorry I was out when you phoned. I did phone you back later that evening but there was no reply.'

'I was at a dental meeting.'

I wanted to ask her about her evening out and the boy she'd been with but I decided against it. At least she seemed quite amicable and made no mention of our disagreement. In fact, it was almost as if she had completely forgotten about it.

'Can I see you this weekend?' I asked tentatively.

'I'd like that, Justin. When did you have in mind?'

'What are you doing this morning?'

'I'm just about to go shopping but I won't be very long and I'm coming your way. Would you like me to call in at your cottage? I could be there by about eleven o'clock.'

'That would be marvellous.'

'See you later then, bye.'

So far, so good; perhaps she had forgiven me. She had seemed very displeased when she walked out on me but perhaps she was the type to forgive and forget easily. People with auburn hair tend to have a reputation for being fiery but often that means that they blow and then quickly forget it and don't hold grudges. I didn't know her well enough to say whether this applied to Harriet but I certainly wanted to find out. I watched the clock anxiously, waiting for her to turn up on my doorstep so that I could put phase two of my plan into operation.

It was almost quarter past eleven when I saw her arrive in Ellie May. I ran out to meet her and took her in my arms and kissed her. She returned my kiss eagerly and I immediately felt that she was as pleased as I was that we were back together. She looked more stunningly beautiful than ever and I knew then that I must never again get into a situation that might tear us apart. I had come to realise that life without her was unthinkable.

I took her inside and made her some coffee and we sat together on the sofa. My palms became clammy and my stomach started to turn somersaults as I got myself ready for my next move. I had been rehearsing whilst waiting for her to arrive but all my preparation proved worthless because logical thought was brought to an abrupt halt by sheer nerves. I almost bottled out completely and it was as if some external force took over and caused me to blurt out clumsily, 'Harriet, will you marry me?'

Her face conveyed surprise, or was it shock? Or could it be horror? I couldn't tell but I was painfully aware that I was making a complete hash of proposing to her. You're asking her to spend the rest of her life with you for God's sake, I thought to myself, not asking her to give you a lift into town.

I moved closer to her and took hold of her hand. 'Harriet, I love you and I want to be with you always. Will you do me the honour of becoming my wife?'

I still couldn't read her expression and just as she seemed to be about to say something the telephone rang. 'Damn,' I exclaimed. 'What a time for someone to ring.'

'You'd better answer it, Justin,' said Harriet quietly. 'It might be important.'

What could be more important than asking you to marry me? I said to myself, then it occurred to me that perhaps she simply wanted more time to think before giving me her answer. Perhaps the telephone call had provided her with a golden opportunity to prepare her reasons for turning me down. I'm sure she wasn't expecting me to propose and it must have come as a great surprise to her. It wasn't unreasonable for her to need time to think about it.

I picked up the handset. 'Hello,' I snapped.

'Ah Mr Derwent, it's Mr Froy here. I'm sorry to trouble you at home but it's rather urgent.'

'How did you get my home number?' I demanded.

'Mr Padginton gave it to me. I phoned the practice and spoke to him but he said he'd just closed the surgery and was on his way out. Apparently he's going to Wales and won't be back until Sunday night. I told him that I needed urgent attention so he gave me your number.'

'Thanks a bunch, Spencer,' I mumbled. 'So what is it that's so important that it forced you to contact me on my Saturday off and couldn't have waited until Monday?'

'I've got a loose tooth that needs to come out.'

'Is it painful?'

'Not too bad.'

'Then it can wait until Monday. If the pain gets worse take some pain killers and come and see me on Monday morning.'

'Ah well the thing is, Mr Derwent, I'm leaving for Ireland in an hour's time and I want to throw the tooth into the Irish Sea.'

I groaned but I didn't feel I had the strength to resist any more. I think I had got myself in such an emotional state over Harriet that all my energy had drained out of me. 'All right, Mr Froy,' I replied feebly, 'can you be at the surgery in twenty minutes?'

'I sure can, Mr Derwent and thank you so much.'

I put the phone down and turned to face Harriet whose expression still gave me no clue as to how she would respond to my proposal. I went back to the sofa, sat down beside her and anxiously waited for her to speak to me.